T0133346

Studien zur Mustererkennung

herausgegeben von:

Prof. Dr.-Ing. Heinrich Niemann
Prof. Dr.-Ing. Elmar Nöth

Bibliografische Information der Deutschen Nationalbibliothek

Die Deutsche Nationalbibliothek verzeichnet diese Publikation in der
Deutschen Nationalbibliografie; detaillierte bibliografische Daten sind
im Internet über http://dnb.d-nb.de abrufbar.

©Copyright Logos Verlag Berlin GmbH 2019

Alle Rechte vorbehalten.

ISBN 978-3-8325-4937-4
ISSN 1617-0695

Logos Verlag Berlin GmbH
Comeniushof
Gubener Str. 47
10243 Berlin
Tel.: +49 030 42 85 10 90
Fax: +49 030 42 85 10 92
INTERNET: http://www.logos-verlag.de

3-D Imaging of Coronary Vessels Using C-arm CT

3D-Bildgebung der Koronargefäße mit C-Bogen CT

Der Technischen Fakultät
der Friedrich-Alexander-Universität
Erlangen-Nürnberg

zur

Erlangung des Doktorgrades Dr.-Ing.

vorgelegt von

Chris Schwemmer

aus

Nürnberg

Als Dissertation genehmigt
von der Technischen Fakultät
der Friedrich-Alexander-Universität Erlangen-Nürnberg

Tag der mündlichen Prüfung: 29.03.2019
Vorsitzender des Promotionsorgans: Prof. Dr.-Ing. R. Lerch
Gutachter: Prof. Dr.-Ing. J. Hornegger
     Prof. F. Noo, PhD
     Prof. Dr.-Ing. M. Grzegorzek

Abstract

Cardiovascular disease has become the number one cause of death worldwide. Its prevention, diagnosis and therapy are therefore highly important topics in today's clinical practice and research. For the diagnosis and therapy of coronary artery disease, interventional C-arm-based fluoroscopy is an imaging method of choice. It delivers 2-D X-ray images from almost arbitrary directions, but a 2-D projection image is naturally limited in its depiction of complex spatial relations. While the C-arm systems are capable of rotating around the patient and thus allow a CT-like 3-D image reconstruction, their long rotation time of about five seconds leads to strong motion artefacts in 3-D coronary artery imaging. Several methods to estimate the coronary motion and compensate for it during 3-D image reconstruction can be found in the literature. All have their specific properties, advantages and disadvantages, which are discussed in the first part of this thesis.

Then, a novel method is introduced that is based on a 2-D–2-D image registration algorithm, henceforth called RMC (Registration-based Motion Compensation). It is embedded in an iterative algorithm for motion estimation and compensation. RMC does not require any complex segmentation or user interaction and is thus fully automatic, which is a very desirable feature for interventional applications. Motion estimation and compensation becomes more difficult when projection data from the whole heart cycle is used from the beginning. RMC overcomes this by successively increasing the utilised amount of projections in a bootstrapping process.

Throughout the remainder of this thesis, RMC is first evaluated in a simulation study using a simple numerical phantom, then on the publicly available CAVAREV platform (employing an anthropomorphic phantom), and finally in a study using 58 human clinical datasets. Through the simulation study, approximations for the inherent error of the investigated algorithms were established. In addition, evidence that the missing depth information of a 2-D motion model is not a limiting factor for coronary artery imaging was found. The CAVAREV experiments investigated the effect of different filter kernel choices during the execution of RMC. For the quantitative evaluation on human clinical data, a new software called CoroEval was introduced to the scientific community.

Overall, it could be shown from both the quantitative results as well as the human observer ratings that RMC can be successfully applied to a large set of clinical data without user interaction or parameter changes, and with a high robustness against initial 3-D image quality, while delivering results that are at least up to the current state of the art, and better in many cases.

Kurzfassung

Kardiovaskuläre Erkrankungen sind inzwischen die häufigsten Todesursachen weltweit. Ihre Vorbeugung, Diagnose und Therapie sind daher in der heutigen klinischen Forschung und Praxis von großer Bedeutung. Für die Diagnose und Therapie der koronaren Herzerkrankung ist die interventionelle, C-Bogen-basierte Fluoroskopie eine bildgebende Methode der Wahl. Sie liefert zweidimensionale Röntgenbilder aus beinahe beliebigen Blickrichtungen. Jedoch sind 2d-Projektionsbilder in ihren Möglichkeiten begrenzt, komplexe räumliche Beziehungen darzustellen. Auch wenn C-Bogen-Systeme in der Lage sind, um den Patienten herum zu rotieren, und damit eine CT-artige dreidimensionale Bildrekonstruktion erlauben, führt ihre lange Rotationszeit von ca. fünf Sekunden zu starken Bewegungsartefakten bei der 3d-Bildgebung der Koronararterien. In der Literatur finden sich verschiedene Methoden, die Bewegung der Koronargefäße zu schätzen und während der 3d-Bildrekonstruktion zu kompensieren. Ihre spezifischen Eigenschaften, Vor- und Nachteile, werden im ersten Teil dieser Arbeit besprochen.

Anschließend wird eine neue Methode vorgestellt, die auf einer 2d–2d-Bildregistrierung basiert, im folgenden RMC (Registration-based Motion Compensation, registrierungsbasierte Bewegungskompensation) genannt. Sie ist in einen iterativen Algorithmus zur Bewegungsschätzung und -kompensation eingebettet. RMC benötigt keine komplexen Segmentierungen oder Benutzereingaben und ist daher vollautomatisch, eine sehr willkommene Eigenschaft im interventionellen Umfeld. Werden von Anfang an Projektionsbilder aus dem gesamten Herzzyklus verwendet, wird die Bewegungsschätzung und -kompensation schwieriger. Dies wird bei RMC dadurch gelöst, dass nach und nach die Anzahl der verwendeten Projektionen in einem Bootstrap-Verfahren erhöht wird.

Im restlichen Teil dieser Arbeit wird RMC zuerst in einer Simulationsstudie mit Hilfe eines einfachen numerischen Phantoms, dann auf der öffentlichen CAVAREV-Plattform (die ein anthropomorphisches Phantom verwendet), und schließlich in einer Studie mit 58 klinischen Patienten-Datensätzen evaluiert. Im Rahmen der Simulationsstudie konnten Näherungen für den Eigenfehler der untersuchten Algorithmen bestimmt werden. Weiterhin wurde aufgezeigt, dass die fehlende Tiefeninformation eines 2d-Bewegungsmodells bei der Koronarbildgebung kein limitierender Faktor ist. Die CAVAREV-Experimente untersuchten den Einfluss verschiedener Filterkerne während der Ausführung von RMC. Zur Unterstützung der quantitativen Auswertung der klinischen Daten wurde eine neue Software namens CoroEval eingeführt.

Insgesamt konnte mit den quantitativen Ergebnissen und den Bewertungen eines menschlichen Beobachters gezeigt werden, dass RMC erfolgreich und mit hoher Robustheit gegenüber der initialen 3d-Bildqualität auf eine große Menge klinischer Daten angewandt werden kann, und dabei weder eine Benutzerinteraktion noch eine Parameteränderungen nötig sind. Die dabei erzielten Ergebnisse entsprechen mindestens dem aktuellen Stand der Technik und übertreffen ihn in vielen Fällen.

Acknowledgement

None of us is as smart as all of us. – Ken Blanchard

A large body of work such as a PhD project can only be accomplished in a good, collaborative environment. I am very grateful to have been in such an environment for the past (not so) few years and would like to express my thanks to each and every one who was a part of this journey. In particular:

Prof. Dr.-Ing. Joachim Hornegger, who has supported and encouraged me since I was a student in the Pattern Recognition lecture of 2006. His passion for medical image processing was what made me choose my focus of work, and I have never regretted it ever since. The focus on team play and networking in his lab have allowed me to spend a year abroad in two countries. Thank you for the opportunity to work on this project, many discussions – and constructive disagreements, for bringing together so many fine people at the LME, and for always finding a way to make great things happen.

Dr. Günter Lauritsch, for being a fantastic industry advisor. Endless hours of discussions, brainstormings and proofreading show his dedication to his work, which I had the honour of being part of for three years. Also, there is no more thorough paper draft review than his! Thank you for your patience and kindness, which made those years not only productive, but also thoroughly enjoyable. Thank you as well for many a great walk, be it over mountains, in the woods, or just around the block.

Prof. Dr.-Ing. Andreas Maier, currently acting head of the LME, who already started being my mentor during our time together at Stanford University in 2010. He lead the reconstruction group at the LME with passion and dedication, always being a source of inspiration. Thank you for your support and encouragement, and always having some Good News™.

Prof. Frédéric Noo, PhD, for bringing together all the great people in CT reconstruction for the CT Meeting conferences in Salt Lake City. Those meetings were definitely among the highlights of this project, both scientifically and socially speaking. And certainly a large part of the credit for that goes to the conference host. I am honoured to have you on my committee.

Prof. Dr.-Ing. Marcin Grzegorzek, for accepting to write a third review on very short notice and submitting that review in a phenomenally short time. And, together with PD Dr. med. Harald Rittger, for being on my committee and patiently enduring the search for a defence date, even though we had not had any contact before that.

Many thanks to my colleagues at the LME and at AX (now AT), for fruitful scientific discussion, enjoyable teamwork, and good times outside of work. Special thanks to Wilhelm Haas, Hannes Hofmann, Dr. Matthias John, Dr.-Ing. Markus Kaiser, Dr.-Ing. Marcus Prümmer and Dr. Bernhard Scholz. Also to my working student Albrecht Kleinfeld, who was a tremendous help in performing experiments and collecting data. And to my current colleagues at CT, for gentle encouragement to finally finish this work.

Dr.-Ing. Christopher Rohkohl, for his guidance, support and friendship – and for always being a good sport in the challenge for the best motion estimation algorithm.

Dr.-Ing. Christoph Forman, with whom I had the pleasure of studying and working together for over ten years now. And who has become a very good friend indeed. Thank you for mutual support, good cooking and a great time!

Dr.-Ing. Kerstin Müller, my self-declared "reconstruction twin". Not only for being a wonderful desk neighbour and great colleague, but also for becoming a dear friend. Both of us left our fingerprints in the other's work – finding a place for Subtract-and-Shift being one of the highlights for me. Thank you for making many a day not only bearable but thoroughly enjoyable, including our dinner-rounds with Christoph and our conference trips together. I do sincerely hope one does not only meet twice in life!

Finally, I am indebted to my family for their patience, support and care. Especially during the writing phase, which certainly was a difficult time. Thank you so much for always having my back! And to my girlfriend Mareike, not only for your love and understanding, but for pushing me through to get it done.

Forchheim, 28.04.2019   Chris Schwemmer

Contents

Introduction

Cardiovascular disease (CVD) is the main cause of death worldwide, having surpassed infectious diseases even in many less-wealthy countries in recent times [Moza 15, Worl 17, Wilk 17]. In Europe alone, over 3.9 million deaths a year (about 45 %) are attributed to CVD [Wilk 17]. The estimated cost for the European Union is about € 210 billion each year, over 50 % of which are due to healthcare expenses. Separating out stroke-related mortality, coronary heart disease (CHD) remains the single most common cause of death in Europe: 19–20 % of men and women die from coronary heart disease [Wilk 17]. Reducing this huge economic and social burden is an important and multi-faceted task. On the one hand, CHD has many well-known *modifiable* risk factors like smoking, obesity, physical inactivity, (mal-)nutrition, or even air pollution [Perk 12, Aren 15, Ding 15, Newb 15]. That means that a large amount of CHD-related morbidity and mortality can be prevented by lifestyle changes. On the other hand, for those endangered or already affected by CHD, efficient diagnosis and treatment options are key to limit personal suffering as well as the impact on healthcare expenses.

Early on, good risk stratification can save low-risk patients from unnecessary diagnostic procedures or even over-treatment [Wils 98, Conr 03, Hech 15]. At the same time, (potentially asymptomatic) medium- to high-risk patients can be detected and referred for further, imaging-based diagnosis and tailored treatment. When it comes to coronary imaging, invasive 2-D coronary angiography is still considered the gold standard [Krak 04, Mark 10, Hamm 11], although X-ray computed tomography (CT) and magnetic resonance imaging (MRI) have been able to gain more ground in recent times. The superior spatial resolution combined with target-specific contrasting, "live" view of the patient situation, and the possibility of immediate treatment are the strongest factors in favour of invasive coronary angiography. On the other hand, there is a distinct lack of 3-D information. This shortcoming can e.g. lead to a misjudgement of bifurcation angles or stenosis grades, or incorrect stent sizing [Gree 04, Goll 07, Carr 09, Camp 14]. Therefore, the lack of 3-D information is often compensated for by pre-procedural CT imaging or multiple different imaging angu-

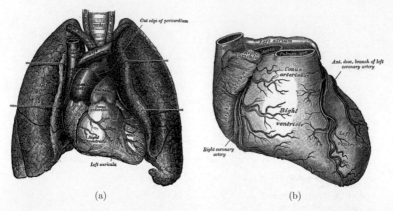

(a)   (b)

Figure 1.1: Anatomy of the human heart. (a) Anterior view of the heart and its surroundings within the thorax. (b) Detailed view of the coronary arteries. Both drawings taken from [Gray 00].

lations during the invasive procedure. The latter is a time-, radiation- and contrast agent-consuming process that also relies on the operator's spatial sense, since the individual 2-D images have to be assembled to a mental picture of the 3-D coronary anatomy [Gree 04]. While there is a possibility to perform CT-like 3-D imaging within an interventional setting, the relatively slow rotation time of angiography systems poses a huge problem for cardiac applications. During a typical acquisition time of 4–5 seconds, a patient's heart may beat 4–10 times. But conventional 3-D reconstruction algorithms expect a static state of the imaged structure throughout all acquired projections. The result of a straight-forward acquisition and reconstruction is therefore not of diagnostical use due to an abundance of motion artefacts and image blur. The goal of this work is to investigate motion estimation and compensation methods integrated into the image reconstruction process. The aim is to bring 3-D imaging of coronary vessels to the interventional suite and validate the resulting methods on a large base of human clinical data.

In the remainder of this chapter, first a short background on anatomy and physiology specific to the coronary system is given. Then, in Section 1.2, potential applications for interventional 3-D cardiac vasculature imaging are motivated. In Section 1.3, the 3-D acquisition protocol that was used for all clinical acquisitions in this work is introduced. Finally, the contributions of this thesis to the progress of research are summarised in Section 1.4 and an outline of the remaining chapters is given in Section 1.5.

1.1   Anatomical and Physiological Background

Anatomy

The human heart is a hollow, muscular organ that is located behind the sternum. It is framed laterally by the lung and sits atop the diaphragm (cf. Fig. 1.1a, diaphragm is the lower image border). The heart's main purpose, pumping blood through the body, is achieved by the interplay of its four chambers – two atria and two ventricles. The right atrium and ventricle drive the pulmonary circulation, moving de-oxygenated blood from the body to the lung. The left atrium and ventricle drive the body's main circulation, which is reflected by the substantially thicker and more muscular walls of the left ventricle. Although the heart's chambers are filled with blood, their walls are too thick to allow for sufficient perfusion of the muscular tissue. Therefore, blood supply for the heart muscles is provided by the coronary arteries (cf. Fig. 1.1b). They originate from the coronary ostia located in the aortic root, close to the aortic valve. Although coronary anatomy varies widely among individuals, the most common configuration shall be discussed here and in the remainder of this work. From the aortic root, two main stems arise: The left coronary artery (LCA), mainly supplying the left heart, and the right coronary artery (RCA), mainly supplying the right heart. The LCA soon branches into the left anterior descending (LAD) and left circumflex (LCX) artery. Typically, the coronary branches that are visible in angiographic images are between ∼1 and 4.5 mm in diameter [Dodg 92]. Further details on the most commonly visible coronary branches are provided in Chapter 7.

Physiology

Coronary heart disease, also called coronary artery disease or syndrome, is a common manifestation of arteriosclerosis. It can appear in a stable, gradually progressing form, or as an acute form [Hamm 11, Mont 13]. The stable form is often characterised by well-known symptoms like shortness of breath or chest pain, especially after physical exercise. On the other hand, for the acute form, about 50 % of deaths "occur in previously asymptomatic patients" [Beck 08]. In both forms, arteriosclerotic plaque builds up in the coronary arteries, leading to an increasingly narrow vessel lumen and therefore an under-perfusion of the heart tissue that is fed by this coronary. In the acute form, plaque that has built up in a larger diameter section of the vessel is loosened and washed downwards until it completely blocks the vessel [Hamm 11].

Over each heart cycle, the interplay of the contracting and relaxing muscles of the four chambers results in a characteristic motion pattern of the heart. Since the coronary vessels are directly attached to the surface of the heart, their motion follows the same pattern. By attaching electrodes to the chest, an electrocardiogram (ECG) can be measured. It describes the electrical signals that govern that heart's beating. There is a very close, although not perfect, correlation between the ECG signal and the actual mechanical motion [Desj 04]. Figure 1.2 shows the relation between ECG signal and physiological events during one full heart cycle. The most obvious feature of an ECG signal is the QRS complex, with its characteristic, strong R peak. It is easy to detect computationally and therefore used for most ECG-correlated image

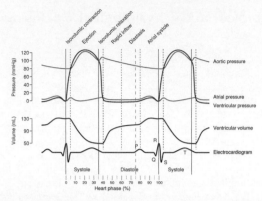

Figure 1.2: The human heart cycle and its temporal relationship between physiological events and ECG signal.
Original image "Wiggers Diagram"[1] © Daniel Chang, MD; DestinyQx; Konrad Conrad. Modified and used under http://creativecommons.org/licenses/by-sa/2.5.

processing. By defining a percentage scale between two consecutive R peaks, the relative distance between the R peaks shall be called *heart phase*. It is shown in light blue at the bottom of Figure 1.2. For the following description of physiological events, we shall concentrate on the left heart. The principles are the same for the right heart, and motion happens simultaneously. The QRS complex triggers the contraction of the blood-filled ventricles, called (ventricular) systole. The mechanical contraction starts around the R peak (0 / 100 % heart phase), but the actual ejection phase begins at the end of the S wave: When the ventricular pressure rises above the aortic pressure, the aortic valve opens (~5 % heart phase). The blood in the left ventricle is then rapidly ejected into the aorta. Systole ends around 35 % heart phase, when the ventricular pressure falls below the aortic pressure and the aortic valve closes again. At the end of the T wave (~40 % heart phase), ventricular pressure drops below atrial pressure and the mitral valve opens, marking the start of the filling phase. The range between 60 and 80 % heart phase is a period of relatively few motion and is called diastasis. It ends when the P wave triggers atrial contraction, filling the ventricle fully and leading up to a new heart cycle. Considering the described motion pattern, it becomes obvious that ECG-correlated imaging or reconstruction should focus on either end-systole (30–40 % heart phase) or mid- to end-diastole / diastasis (60–80 % heart phase). Although the length of diastasis varies with heart rate [Husm 07], it is generally the longer time window and therefore commonly used [Lu 01, Ruzs 09]. The end-diastolic 75 % time point that was successfully used in previous work [Desj 04, Rohk 11] as well as this work [Schw 13b, Schw 13a] is marked with a light blue dashed line in Figure 1.2.

---

[1]http://commons.wikimedia.org/wiki/File:Wiggers_Diagram.svg

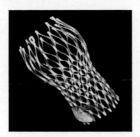 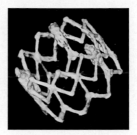

Figure 1.3: Two in-vivo trans-catheter aortic valves reconstructed with the methods presented in this work.

1.2   Potential Applications for Interventional 3-D Cardiac Vasculature Imaging

Although invasive 2-D coronary angiography is considered the gold standard for imaging the coronary arteries, the lack of 3-D information can lead to longer procedure times, increased radiation and contrast burden, or even misinterpretations and possibly wrong decisions. For complex vessel topologies, a 3-D reconstruction of the cardiac vasculature could provide procedure planning and roadmapping without the need for repeated 2-D acquisitions from different angulations [Wink 03, Madd 04, Goll 07, Scho 09, Hett 10, Morr 15]. In addition to that, optimal viewing angles can be calculated from a 3-D coronary tree that minimise foreshortening during fluoroscopy [Chen 02, Eng 13]. When the 3-D image is registered to the current fluoroscopic angulation, live procedure guidance could possibly be achieved without application of further contrast agent [Turg 05, Garc 09]. If motion information is available, this guidance overlay can even be adjusted according to the current heart phase. Instead of registration to the fluoroscopic image, a fusion with intra-vascular ultrasound (IVUS) or optical coherence tomography (OCT) data is also an option, complementing the 3-D information with the superior plaque assessment of these modalities. Finally, stenosis quantification from a single angiographic projection can lead to wrong diagnoses due to the non-circular cross-section of coronary vessels in addition to foreshortening [Madd 04]. Therefore, a quantitatively reliable 3-D reconstruction of the coronary tree would be highly desirable.

Although the acquisition protocol described in the next section is tailored to coronary artery imaging, two further potential applications of this work shall be mentioned here. For bi-ventricular pacemaker implantation, a 3-D reconstruction of the coronary sinus (i.e. veins) can help to reduce procedure time, radiation and contrast burden, as well as have the potential to improve outcomes [Gutl 11, Ma 12, Dori 13]. Though not further discussed in this work, [Gutl 11] showed that with a different contrast injection scheme, sufficient opacification can be achieved for motion-compensated 3-D reconstruction of the coronary sinus to be feasible.

Trans-catheter aortic valve implantation (TAVI) procedures have seen a strong increase recently [Egge 16]. The planning of such procedures is a strong domain of

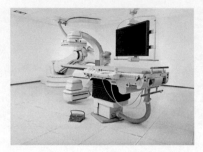

Figure 1.4: An Artis zeego robotic C-arm system (Siemens Healthcare GmbH, Forchheim, Germany, image used with kind permission).

Table 1.1: Parameters of the employed acquisition protocol.

Acquisition type	single-rotation, circ. trajectory	Source-detector-dist.	~120 cm
Contrasting	at coronary ostium, 1–2 ml/s	Source-isocentre-dist.	~80 cm
Rotation time	5 s	Fan angle	20°
# Proj. images	133	Cone angle	7°
Angular spacing	1.5°	Angle covered	200°
Detector frame rate	30 / s	Focal spot size	0.6 mm
Detector size	40 × 30 cm	kVp	~70–100
Proj. image size	1240 × 960 pixels	Dose / image	0.36 µGy
Pixel size	0.308 mm (isotropic)		

non-invasive CT coronary angiography [Ache 12] and will most probably remain so. But during the procedure there might arise situations where current 3-D information becomes helpful. For example, new devices are entering the market that allow to retract and re-position the valve after its initial deployment [Serr 13]. The 3-D relation of such a valve to calcium deposits or anatomy could be gained from a 3-D reconstruction. The principle feasibility of applying the results of this work to implanted TAVI devices is shown empirically in Figure 1.3.

The potential applications discussed in this section are the principal motivation for this work and the ones closest to a direct application in clinical routine. Two further applications, namely motion analysis and virtual fractional flow reserve (FFR) calculation, are shortly discussed in the outlook (Section 8.2.2).

1.3 C-arm 3-D Acquisition Protocol for Coronary Vasculature

Invasive coronary angiography is performed in an interventional suite equipped with a C-arm device (cf. Fig. 1.4). Such devices are basically an X-ray source and a detector mounted on a C-shaped frame that can be moved more or less arbitrarily in space. The intention of this setup is the quick availability of different imaging angulations during the procedure. By positioning the C-arm accordingly, the interventionalist can get the best possible view of the advancing catheter and the patient's anatomy. At the same time, due to the open frame of the system, the patient remains accessible during the whole procedure. This is in contrast to MR- or CT-based interventions, where patient access is restricted by the gantry bore. During the 1990s, interest turned towards 3-D imaging with C-arm devices [Roug 93, Sain 94, Fahr 97]. Since these systems allow a rotational acquisition on a circular trajectory around the patient [Tomm 98], the idea of CT-like imaging in an interventional setting is a natural extension of the C-arm's 2-D capabilities. In practice, many obstacles like mechanical stability, photon scatter and more needed to be addressed [Zell 05, Orth 09, Stro 09, Wall 09]. Today, all major C-arm manufacturers provide 3-D options for their devices, marketed as e.g. DynaCT (Siemens Healthcare GmbH, Forchheim, Germany), XperCT (Philips Healthcare, Andover, MA, USA), Innova CT (GE Healthcare, Chalfont St. Giles, UK) or Infinix (Toshiba Corporation, Minato/Tokyo, Japan).

Still, due to the slow rotation speed of the devices, only 3-D imaging of static objects is of practical clinical relevance today. For moving objects like cardiac vasculature, a motion compensation like the one discussed in this work needs to be employed. While there are other possibilities of overcoming heart motion-related artefacts, like rapid pacing or stopping the heart altogether, patient safety and comfort are severely affected by these. Also, multiple-rotation, ECG-triggered acquisition delivers too much radiation dose to the patient. Therefore, the acquisition protocol employed in this work relies on a five second single-rotation scan under breath-hold and natural heart rhythm (i.e. no pacing or medication), with synchronous recording of the ECG signal. This protocol was already successfully used in [Rohk 11].

A distinctive advantage of invasive coronary angiography is the ability to directly administer contrast agent to a target vessel. Thus, a catheter is placed at either the left or right coronary ostium and contrast agent is injected throughout the acquisition with a flow rate of 1–2 ml/s, resulting in a total contrast burden of ∼10 ml for the acquisition. CT coronary angiography on the other hand relies on intravenous contrast administration, necessitating a larger contrast agent burden to achieve sufficient vessel opacification: Typical total contrast agent amounts for CT coronary angiography are between 60 and 100 ml [Schr 08]. Since typical X-ray contrast agents are nephrotoxic [McCu 08], a small usage is a distinct advantage. The disadvantage of the selective contrasting employed here is that always only one side of the coronary tree is visible, depending on which ostium the catheter was placed at.

The effective dose delivered to the patient with this protocol is estimated to be around 1–2 mSv. Dose measurements for a similar protocol were reported with 3.31 mSv [Hohl 08]. That protocol used a detector entrance dose of 0.54 µGy per image and acquired 248 projection images in total. Since the protocol used for this work employs 2/3 less dose per image and acquires ∼50 % less projection images, 1–2 mSv seem to be a realistic dose estimate. For comparison, CT coronary angiography delivers 5–20 mSv [Schr 08], down to less than 1 mSv under ideal circumstances [Hell 14, Mors 14].

All clinical datasets in this work were acquired on Artis zee and zeego systems (Siemens Healthcare GmbH, Forchheim, Germany) using flat panel detectors with a size of 40×30 cm. An overview of the technical protocol details is given in Table 1.1.

1.4   Scientific Contribution

2-D–2-D Motion Estimation and Compensation

A novel projection-based method for motion estimation and compensation of coronary vasculature was introduced. It is based on a multi-resolution, deformable registration in projection space and does not require complex pre-processing steps like explicit coronary segmentation. In addition, the method is fully automatic. Due to the lower complexity of a 2-D motion model, more control points than in a comparable 3-D motion model can be used, leading to a higher spatial resolution of the motion vector field.

First, the method was used for residual motion compensation in ECG-gated reconstruction. This work was published at an international conference [Schw 12] and in a peer-reviewed journal article [Schw 13b]. Later, it could be shown how to extend the gating window size up to 100 % of the available projection data by a bootstrapping-like approach, which increases signal strength. These results were presented at another international conference [Schw 13a].

Clinical Data Evaluation of Motion Compensation Algorithms

A software utility to support the structured and repeatable evaluation of image quality metrics on clinical 3-D coronary artery reconstructions was developed in a cooperative effort with Christoph Forman and Jens Wetzl. This framework supports data from multiple modalities (currently C-arm CT, CT and MRI) and was released to the public as open source software. A corresponding article was published in a peer-reviewed journal [Schw 14a]. The projection-based motion estimation and compensation method introduced in this work was evaluated both on phantom data and on a large-scale human clinical data pool. A summary of the results was presented at an international conference [Schw 14b].

During the work on the numerical phantom study (cf. Chapter 4), contributions to the CONRAD framework were made with regard to efficient B-spline evaluation [Maie 12] and the phantom framework itself [Maie 13]. Additionally, work on artefact reduction by removal of high-density objects [Schw 10], while turning out not to be useful for coronary vasculature reconstruction, was successfully employed in reconstruction of the cardiac chambers [Mull 14b, Mull 14c] and fiducial marker removal [Berg 14]. Finally, a patent on virtual FFR computation employs the results of this work for the reconstruction of the coronary tree [Laur 15].

In total, the results of this work were part of five international conference presentations [Schw 12, Schw 13a, Berg 14, Mull 14b, Schw 14b], five journal articles [Maie 12, Schw 13b, Maie 13, Mull 14c, Schw 14a] and one patent [Laur 15].

1.5   Outline

In this section, a chapter-wise outline of this thesis is given. It serves as a structured overview of the upcoming chapters.

Chapter 2 – State of the Art

In Chapter 2, the state of the art in cardiovascular imaging with C-arm CT is reviewed. First, model-based approaches are discussed that result in a centreline and/or
lumen model of the coronary tree. The main focus of the chapter is on tomographic
methods that deliver a 3-D image with voxel intensities corresponding to the X-ray
absorption of tissue. These methods can be further divided into iterative and analytical approaches. Both are introduced, again with a focus on analytical methods.
The most straight forward application of motion compensation to analytical reconstruction is by ECG gating. Unfortunately, this does not result in sufficient image
quality for a final clinically useful image. But several studies have shown that these
gated reconstructions serve as good initial estimates for further motion estimation
algorithms, which are reviewed accordingly. The NOPMEC algorithm, which is used as
a reference for comparison in further chapters, is introduced in more detail. Finally,
the body of work on the evaluation of motion-compensated coronary reconstructions
is reviewed before the chapter is concluded with a summary.

Chapter 3 – 2-D–2-D Motion Estimation and Compensation

The main algorithmic contribution of this work is presented in Chapter 3. The
method uses an initial, ECG-gated reconstruction as a reference template for motion
estimation. It starts with a small ECG gating window to increase temporal resolution.
Undersampling artefacts are reduced by a heuristic streak-reduction technique. Using
a bootstrapping-like method, the gating window size is gradually increased to up to
100 % of the available projection data. After introducing the motion estimation
and compensation algorithms and all its components, the chapter continues with a
complexity analysis of the method. Since the same parameter set is used throughout
all following chapters, these parameters are presented and motivated subsequently.
Finally, a short summary is given.

Chapter 4 – Numerical Phantom Study

The first evaluation chapter is concerned with a numerical simulation study. A simple
numerical sphere phantom is introduced and the generated test datasets and evaluation metrics are described. A qualitative and quantitative analysis of the results
is given. By using both a static and dynamic phantom in different sphere configurations, a baseline error for the investigated motion estimation and compensation
algorithms is established.

Chapter 5 – CAVAREV Simulation Study

Following the simple phantom study, Chapter 5 covers the evaluation using the public
CAVAREV platform. This platform provides projection image data from an anthropomorphic phantom that simulates a beating heart with selectively contrasted coronary
arteries. It also provides evaluation metrics and a publicly available ranking. First,
the platform and its datasets and metrics, as well as the experimental setup are

introduced. The results are presented and analysed. The validity of the parameter choices and the general applicability of the presented algorithm to cardiac vasculature reconstruction is demonstrated by these results.

Chapter 6 – Human Clinical Study – Quantitative Evaluation

Chapter 6 presents the quantitative part of an evaluation study on human clinical data. For this evaluation, a software tool called CoroEval was developed. This software is introduced and validated in the first part of the chapter. Next an outline of the patient population is given and the study design, including evaluation protocol and statistical analysis, is presented. A detailed analysis of the quantitative results and algorithm runtime behaviour follows. It is shown that the algorithm introduced in this work can be successfully applied to a large set of clinical data without the need for an adjustment of any parameters and with a high robustness against the quality of the initial reconstruction.

Chapter 7 – Human Clinical Study – Qualitative Evaluation

In the second part of the study on human clinical data, the qualitative evaluation is presented. A non-blinded human observer study with one anatomically trained observer was carried out during the course of this work. The rating scheme used is introduced first. Then the results and image examples are presented and analysed. The overall findings of the quantitative evaluation are confirmed and more insight in the underlying reasons for previous observations is gained.

Chapter 8 – Summary and Outlook

The final chapter concludes this thesis with a summary of the presented research and contributions. An outlook on cardiovascular imaging with C-arm CT is given, including limitations and optimisation potentials of the introduced method, as well as a short review of possible future applications for interventional cardiovascular imaging.

CHAPTER 2

State of the Art

In this chapter, the state of the art on reconstructing the coronary artery tree from interventional C-arm angiography data is presented. This topic has been approached from various angles, depending on acquisition protocol, motion handling, and desired reconstruction result. Approaches concerned with tomographic reconstruction from rotational angiography ("C-arm CT") will receive the main focus here. In the literature, several reviews can be found that also cover the other approaches in greater detail, e.g. [Chen 09, Scho 09, Rohk 11]. The most recent and also most comprehensive review is [Cime 16]. Their classification scheme for the different types of approaches is also used here.

This thesis assumes a general familiarity of the reader with CT image reconstruction theory. For an excellent introduction into the topic and more detailed background, [Buzu 08] is recommended. The notation used throughout the remainder of this thesis follows the one introduced in [Rohk 11] and is defined in Section 2.3 and Chapter 3.

Some of the first methods for coronary tree reconstruction were not of tomographic nature, but resulted in a centreline and/or lumen model of the tree. Therefore, Section 2.1 introduces these methods and their strengths and limitations. In Section 2.2, tomographic reconstruction methods are discussed, with a focus on analytic reconstruction. One such state-of-the-art algorithm, the NOPMEC algorithm, is introduced in greater detail in Section 2.3, since it will be used as a basis for comparison in the later chapters of this thesis. In Section 2.4, methods for the evaluation of the quality of a coronary reconstruction are discussed. Finally, this chapter is summarised and concluded in Section 2.5.

2.1 Model-based reconstruction

According to [Cime 16], we denote those approaches to be model-based that do not result in a tomographic reconstruction of the coronary tree. That means their result is not a greyscale image, where intensity values correspond to the X-ray absorption of tissue. Instead, these approaches build a 3-D centreline and/or lumen model of the coronary tree. This can actually be a desirable feature of an algorithm, if its result is to be used for further automated processing, where a 3-D model is more useful than an intensity image that needs further segmentation. On the other hand, all information about X-ray absorption from the original acquisition is lost, which precludes the analysis of contrast agent distribution or other grey value-based investigations.

One possibility for a model-based reconstruction is to start with an atlas-based 3-D model of the coronary tree and adapt it to the actual 2-D projection images at hand. Usually, smoothness and topology constraints are employed to avoid a degeneration of the model. So far, all published approaches using this idea require a manual correspondence selection or some other form of interaction for initialisation [Zhu 02, Yang 14, Cong 15]. Another problem of these approaches is the initial 3-D model. The anatomy of coronary trees is highly diverse, even for healthy patients. In diseased patients, occluded arteries, collaterals and previous interventions increase the variability. This means that all assumptions about tree topology limit the applicability of the model. Total freedom, on the other hand, makes models difficult to handle.

Therefore, a second approach to model-based reconstruction starts with a segmentation of 2-D features in the acquired projection data. Such features could be, for example, coronary centrelines or vesselness filter responses (e.g. [Fran 98]). Those features are then back-projected using the acquisition geometry [Chen 00, Blon 06, Fall 08, Yang 09, Ceti 16] or used in another analytical formulation of the reconstruction problem [Keil 09]. One very interesting feature of these approaches is that they can estimate the projection geometry of the acquisition system during reconstruction, since a correspondence of the extracted features from different viewing angles is sought. This simultaneous calibration during reconstruction removes the need for an offline calibration that tomographic reconstruction methods have. On the other hand, the reconstruction problem becomes even more ill-posed, since additional parameters have to be estimated in addition to the coronary tree and its motion. Still, the beforementioned approaches relying on centreline features need a 2-D vessel segmentation, which is known to be a difficult task [Jand 09b]. In addition, a correspondence selection of coronary tree segments from different viewing angles is needed. Either this is performed manually, which is not feasible in an interventional setting for many projection images. Or epipolar constraints with a local search strategy are employed. The output of the centreline-based methods is only a 3-D centreline model at first. To get a 3-D lumen model, a lumen estimation step needs to be added afterwards [Mova 04, Jand 09b]. In contrast, [Jand 09a] back-projected the response of a vesselness filter to avoid both the difficulty of full 2-D centreline segmentation and separate lumen estimation. But they noted an extensive noise in the 3-D vesselness result due to the limited number of projections available [Jand 09a].

2.2   Tomographic reconstruction

Tomographic reconstruction methods result in greyscale images, with a direct correspondence of X-ray absorption to intensity values. As discussed in the previous section, this can give way to further analysis of pathologies. Since no model assumption on the coronary tree is present in most of the tomographic methods, they can implicitly handle any anatomic or pathological configuration. On the other hand, for an explicit model representation of the coronary tree topology and lumen, further segmentation is necessary. Luckily, 3-D segmentation of the coronary artery tree from C-arm CT data is relatively easy compared to 2-D segmentation in the projection images, due to a high vessel-to-background contrast and no overlap between multiple structures. In contrast to the model-based approaches, most of the tomographic methods do not need complex interactive segmentation or correspondence selection steps, which is a very desirable property in the interventional setting. Last, it should also be noted that the resulting CT-like image from these methods has a more natural look compared to the artificial-looking model-based reconstructions, which increases acceptability.

A notable disadvantage of the tomographic reconstruction methods is the need for a well-calibrated acquisition geometry to avoid image artefacts. In addition, while model-based approaches can often be used with very few (down to two) projection images, tomographic approaches by definition need a dedicated rotational angiography acquisition protocol that covers a sufficient angular range with low angular spacing between the acquired projections. During the whole acquisition, a constant contrast opacification of the coronary arteries is necessary to fulfil the assumption of all tomographic algorithms that the same object is observed from all angulations. Finally, owing to the higher number of projections, and the inherent ill-posedness of the reconstruction problem, the computational demand of tomographic methods is generally higher than that of the model-based methods [Cime 16].

2.2.1   Iterative reconstruction

In iterative reconstruction, the reconstruction task is considered as an optimisation problem. Given a 3-D reconstruction, its forward projections using the acquisition geometry should match the original 2-D projection images. The minimisation of the deviations between these forward projections and the original projections is the optimisation problem [Buzu 08]. Generally, due to the overdetermined nature of this problem, the solution is sought iteratively, hence the name of this technique.

How the initial 3-D reconstruction is computed and represented, how forward projections are generated, and how the minimisation problem is solved, varies between implementations. Due to the great flexibility in the concrete implementation of these aspects, there is great freedom for the modelling of physical effects and system constraints in iterative reconstruction. On the other hand, this poses a high computational demand that generally results in longer processing times than for analytic reconstruction methods [Buzu 08].

The initial assumption of iterative reconstruction, that a forward projection of the ideal 3-D reconstruction perfectly matches the original 2-D projection image, is invalid in the presence of motion. If a static 3-D image is reconstructed, it can only match one motion state, which will not be reflected by all of the projection images. This leads to a non-convergence of classical iterative reconstruction methods in the presence of motion. In the literature, three approaches can be found to solve this issue for coronary reconstruction. First, the minimisation strategy can be adapted as in [Hans 08a] by exploiting the sparse nature of the coronary tree and minimising the L_1 norm of the reconstructed image constrained by the deviation between forward projections and original projections. The second approach is an adaption of the forward projector to incorporate a motion model [Blon 04, Scho 07, Hans 09]. This explicitly accounts for motion in the formulation of the optimisation problem, but is again computationally more expensive. However, the ideas underlying these iterative reconstruction methods can also be found in the analytic reconstruction methods discussed below, including the one that is the topic of this work. One could speak of a hybrid approach, where analytical reconstruction is combined with an iterative optimisation of the motion model. Finally, [Taub 16a, Taub 17] recently introduced an approach that applies strictly gated reconstruction (as discussed in the next section) in an iterative reconstruction framework. The objective function contains both a spatial norm (as in [Hans 08a]), as well as a temporal norm that helps offset the disadvantages of strict gating. Its performance on phantom data look promising, but an evaluation on a larger set of clinical data is not available at the time of this writing.

2.2.2 Analytic reconstruction

In analytic reconstruction, as the name suggests, an analytic solution for the reconstruction problem is sought. That means that an explicit function can be given that defines the mapping between the measured projection data and the reconstructed 3-D attenuation values. What it does not mean, is that this function is an exact solution of the reconstruction problem. In fact, the most common family of cone-beam reconstruction algorithms is approximative. All of the approaches discussed in this section are based on the Feldkamp-Davis-Kress (FDK) algorithm [Feld 84]. This algorithm can be very efficiently implemented, especially on massively parallelising hardware like graphics cards [Rohk 09a]. On the other hand, there is very little freedom to account for non-ideal system properties, as their analytical formulation is quite complex. In addition, the approximative nature of the FDK algorithm, combined with the limited angular coverage and large X-ray cone angle of C-arm flat panel systems, leads to an inherent reconstruction error even for a static object [Buzu 08, Stro 09]. Whether this inherent error matters depends on the intended use of the reconstructed images. Especially for high contrast imaging applications like the coronary arteries, it certainly is of lesser concern.

Gated reconstruction

As seen in Section 1.1, there are certain periods of very little heart motion during the end-systole and during diastasis. Therefore, one very obvious approach to reduce the effect of motion on the reconstruction is to perform an ECG-gated reconstruction. If an ECG signal is recorded simultaneously with the acquisition, a retrospective gating of X-ray projection data can be performed: Only images from a specific heart phase contribute to the reconstruction [Desj 04]. However, ECG data does not necessarily correspond to the exact motion state of the heart [Desj 04]. This means ECG-gating will always be imperfect, leading to residual motion. In addition, ECG-gating sparsifies data and therefore reconstruction becomes a strongly ill-posed problem, limiting the quality and usability of the resulting 3-D data. To compensate for this, not a strict gating, but a temporal window with a certain width around the selected motion state is used [Rohk 08b]. The shape of the gating window evolved from a pure nearest-neighbour approach [Schä 06] over cosine-shaped [Schä 06] to the most general power-of-cosine shape [Rohk 08b] that can be parametrised very flexibly.

A wider gating window is desirable to get a high signal-to-noise ratio and little undersampling artefacts, but then the additional residual motion in the gated projection data corrupts image quality. Therefore, gating is a trade-off between undersampling artefacts (narrow gating window) and motion artefacts (wide gating window). There has been some work on an automatic selection of the optimal window size [Lehm 06, Rohk 10a], optimal window centre point [Husm 07] or all of the ECG-gating parameters [Rasc 04, Rasc 06, Rohk 10a]. Still, most published work seems to be using fixed parameters.

If no ECG signal is recorded during the acquisition, research on image-based gating has been performed [Blon 06, Lehm 06, Rohk 08a]. It could be shown that an approximation of the cardiac phase information can be derived from only the projection data. Still, if available, an ECG signal delivers more robust phase information.

Although ECG-gated reconstruction alone does not satisfy state-of-the-art expectations on image quality, it has been shown that such gated reconstructions represent a good initial estimate for further motion-compensated reconstruction methods [Rohk 08b, Rohk 10b, Schw 13a, Schw 13b].

Motion estimation and compensation

In this review, only motion estimation methods will be discussed. It was shown in [Schä 06] that motion-compensated reconstruction can be elegantly integrated into an FDK-type reconstruction algorithm. The motion-compensated reconstruction then almost equals the quality of a static reconstruction if the motion vector field is fully known.

As noted in the previous section, ECG gating alone does not lead to ideal reconstruction results, due to residual motion within the gated data. In addition, as shown in [Rohk 09b], motion compensation ideally should not contain periodicity assumptions to account for irregular heart motion during the acquisition. In contrast, ECG gating always assumes periodicity.

In the literature, several approaches have been proposed to account for residual motion due to non-ideal ECG-gating. A general distinction can be made between those that do a full 3-D motion estimation and compensation, and those that perform a 2-D estimation. In between these two are approaches that compute a 3-D motion vector field by 2-D–3-D registration. Motion compensation using a 3-D motion vector field corrects motion in image space, which allows for the greatest freedom in modelling motion. On the other hand, a full 3-D estimation is a strongly ill-posed problem with high computational demands. Motion periodicity assumptions and/or regularisation are therefore often used [Zeng 05, Hans 09]. [Blon 06] did a two-step approach by first performing a model-based motion estimation and then reconstructing the tomographic image by incorporating the estimated motion into the reconstruction algorithm. [Prum 09, Isol 10, Tang 12] proposed a 3-D–3-D registration-based approach. Generally, only one or two time points during the cardiac cycle allow for the reconstruction of images with sufficient quality. Therefore, a 3-D–3-D registration is a very ill-conditioned problem for motion estimation of coronary arteries. Finally, [Rohk 10b] proposed a method that incorporates the motion estimation and reconstruction problems into one analytic formulation. This leads to a very high-dimensional optimisation problem with high computational demands. By implementing a simple cost function that is easy to compute and integrating it into a highly optimised backprojection operation, they were able to achieve reasonable computation times. This algorithm is introduced in more detail in the next section.

Due to the lack of multiple time points where a 3-D image can be reconstructed, another approach is the calculation of a 3-D motion vector field by 2-D–3-D registration. Only one 3-D image of good quality is needed, which is then forward-projected onto the original projection data. By using a 2-D similarity measure, the 3-D motion vector field is optimised until a good fit is obtained. This approach was presented in [Zeng 05] for respiratory motion. [Scha 07] proposed to register markers on the balloon catheter for registration, which is only possible if such markers are present in the acquired data. In general, the ill-conditioned nature of 2-D–3-D registration results in computationally intensive algorithms and the need for a prior motion estimate. [Rohk 10a] proposed a rigid affine motion model to address these issues, which on the other hand is not able to model the cardiac motion as well as deformable motion models.

2-D motion estimation methods work in projection space. This problem is easier and better conditioned, since the parameter space is of lower dimension and the estimation is performed purely on the input data. Due to possible overlay of structures along the X-ray beam direction, a 2-D method is always only an approximation. All structures along the beam are affected by the same transformation during motion compensation. However, the object of interest here, i.e. contrasted vasculature, is very sparse compared to the image volume. Motion in viewing direction in the range of coronary motion is almost impossible to detect in X-ray projection images. In addition, due to the ECG gating, the residual motion within the gating window can be assumed to be reasonably small. Therefore an approximate 2-D estimation in projection space might be sufficient. This is supported by the findings in [Unbe 15]. The torsional motion of the coronaries cannot be accurately modelled by a 2-D motion model. Still, [Unbe 15] only found a small influence on the reconstruction result even for strong torsional motion in severely diseased patients.

In the literature, a couple of projection-based methods can be found, which are discussed shortly. If landmarks are available in the acquired data (e.g. vascular stents or catheter-based markers), these can be tracked and a landmark-based registration can be performed [Mova 03, Perr 07]. However, the availability of such landmarks cannot be assumed for all data. A model-based learning approach was proposed as another method. A previously learnt model is registered to the actual data [Lebo 11]. This means that an extensive training phase is needed in advance. A method based on registration in projection space was proposed in [Hans 08b]. It requires a segmentation of vasculature centrelines in the acquired projection data, which was already identified as difficult [Jand 09b]. [Tagu 07] proposed a method that employs a block-matching algorithm for 2-D motion estimation in cardiac CT.

Finally, all approaches discussed so far result in one static 3-D reconstruction by default. If a 3-D+time reconstruction is desired, several ideas can be found. The simplest approach is a separate static reconstruction for each cardiac phase [Chen 03, Jand 09b]. This leads to a problem with discontinuities between time points. The introduction of temporal constraints between neighbouring phases could help, e.g. by tree matching [Jand 09b]. Another possibility is the deformation of an initial 3-D reconstruction from a reference heart phase to the target heart phases [Zhu 02, Mull 12]. Temporal smoothness can be ensured there by using a 4-D B-spline-based deformation model [Blon 06, Rohk 09b, Mull 12].

2.3   The nopmec Algorithm

In this section, the NOPMEC (non-periodic motion estimation and compensation) algorithm presented in [Rohk 09b, Rohk 10b, Rohk 11] is introduced in more detail. It is a representative of the group of algorithms employing a full 3-D motion estimation and showed good results in the evaluation of the aforementioned publications. In addition, its implementation is available at the Pattern Recognition Lab. Therefore, all experiments in Chapters 4 – 7 were also performed using the NOPMEC algorithm for a direct comparison of a state-of-the-art algorithm with the results of this work. The description of the algorithm, including notation, follows [Rohk 10b].

Reference image creation

As discussed in the section on ECG-gated reconstruction, such a gated reconstruction is often used as an initial estimate for motion estimation algorithms. Therefore, the NOPMEC algorithm starts with the creation of a reference image f_{REF} by ECG-gated reconstruction. The reference heart phase for this reconstruction is typically placed at the diastasis phase. After reconstruction, f_{REF} is post-processed with a threshold-and-scale operation to only retain high-contrast structures (i.e. contrasted vasculature) and map the remaining intensities to the 8-bit range $[0, 255]$. The intensity mapping can be considered as a data normalisation step. In [Rohk 10b], a manual interaction is proposed to select the optimal threshold and scaling factors. Since manual interaction is not desired, [Rohk 11] propose a threshold based on a certain percentile of the image histogram and linearly scaling the remaining intensities.

Motion model

A time-continuous motion model is employed. Time is represented as the acquisition time of a projection image relative to the duration of the scan. The motion model is described by a function

$$M : \mathbb{N} \times \mathbb{R}^3 \times \mathbb{S} \mapsto \mathbb{R}^3, (i, \boldsymbol{x}, \boldsymbol{s}) \mapsto \boldsymbol{x}' , \tag{2.1}$$

where $\boldsymbol{x} = (x_0, x_1, x_2)^{\mathrm{T}}$ is a voxel coordinate that is mapped to the new position $\boldsymbol{x}'$ by the motion model M at time point i. The vector $\boldsymbol{s}$ contains the motion model parameters. NOPMEC uses a motion model based on cubic B-splines [Unse 99] that is parametrised by a set of $C_s \times C_s \times C_s \times C_t$ control points placed uniformly in space and time. Since the motion model encodes the displacement vectors from $\boldsymbol{x}$ to $\boldsymbol{x}'$, this leads to the practical definition of the NOPMEC motion model as

$$M\left(i, \boldsymbol{x}, \boldsymbol{s}\right) = \boldsymbol{x} + \sum_{j,k,l,t} B_j\left(x_0\right) \cdot B_k\left(x_1\right) \cdot B_l\left(x_2\right) \cdot B_t\left(i\right) \cdot \boldsymbol{s}_{jklt} \ . \tag{2.2}$$

The displacement vectors at the control points are stored in

$$\mathbb{S} = \left\{ \boldsymbol{s}_{jklt} \in \mathbb{R}^3 \,|\, 1 \leq j, k, l \leq C_s, 1 \leq t \leq C_t \right\} \ ,$$

interpolation at points between the control points is carried out using the cubic B-spline basis functions B_j, B_k, B_l and B_t.

According to [Schä 06], once a motion model is established, this allows its integration into the FDK reconstruction formulation, resulting in a motion-compensated backprojection:

$$f\left(\boldsymbol{x}, \boldsymbol{s}\right) = \sum_i w\left(i, M\left(i, \boldsymbol{x}, \boldsymbol{s}\right)\right) \cdot p\left(i, A\left(i, M\left(i, \boldsymbol{x}, \boldsymbol{s}\right)\right)\right) \ , \tag{2.3}$$

where $w : \mathbb{N} \times \mathbb{R}^3 \mapsto \mathbb{R}$ returns the distance weight of the FDK formulation. $p : \mathbb{N} \times \mathbb{R}^2 \mapsto \mathbb{R}$ represents the pre-processed, filtered, and redundancy-weighted projection images, with $p\left(i, \boldsymbol{u}\right)$ returning the value of pixel $\boldsymbol{u}$ of image number i. The perspective projection of voxel $\boldsymbol{x}$ to pixel $\boldsymbol{u}$ at time point / image number i is modelled by $A : \mathbb{N} \times \mathbb{R}^3 \mapsto \mathbb{R}^2, (i, \boldsymbol{x}) \mapsto \boldsymbol{u}$.

Objective function

[Rohk 11] propose to use the joint intensity between the reference reconstruction and the current, motion-compensated reconstruction as the objective function for motion estimation. Thus the search for an optimal parameter set $\hat{\boldsymbol{s}} \in \mathbb{S}$ can be formulated as

$$\hat{\boldsymbol{s}} = \operatorname*{argmin}_{\boldsymbol{s} \in \mathbb{S}} \left(-\sum_{\boldsymbol{x}} f_{\mathrm{REF}}\left(\boldsymbol{x}\right) \cdot f\left(\boldsymbol{x}, \boldsymbol{s}\right) \right) \ . \tag{2.4}$$

Using such a simple objective function allows for a direct calculation of its derivative, which in turn enables the use of standard optimisation techniques to find the optimal parameter set (the derivation is laid out in [Rohk 11]). The downside of this objective function is that it does not consider the context of a voxel like e.g. mutual information or normalised cross-correlation would. In addition, supplementing the objective function with additional constraints or metrics would make its analytical derivation very difficult to impossible, which would then remove the great runtime benefits of the direct integration of motion estimation into the image reconstruction.

The L-BFGS-B algorithm that is used by Rohkohl et al is set to stop the optimisation after $I_{\max}$ iterations.

Parameter selection and runtime considerations

Since the reference reconstruction is by design very sparse, and the objective function is a multiplicative operation, the calculation of the objective function can be optimised heavily by only evaluating the $\sim 2\,‰$ remaining non-zero voxels. In addition, evaluation of the B-spline interpolation, calculation of the objective function, and the calculation of Eq. 2.3 was implemented using GPU acceleration by Rohkohl et al. This results in a reported average runtime of ~ 3 minutes in [Rohk 10b]. The possible matrix size of the result image (e.g. 256^3 voxels) is limited by the memory and computation power of the graphics card, since the evaluation of the objective function has a memory and time complexity proportional to said matrix size.

Regarding the choice of the free parameters of the NOPMEC algorithm, [Rohk 10b] report setting $C_s = 5$, $C_t = 35$ and $I_{\max} = 100$. Due to further practical experience with clinical data, we parametrised the algorithm with $C_s = 6$, $C_t = 67$ and $I_{\max} = 100$ for the experiments in this work. The increased spatial sampling allows the motion model to better capture different motion patterns within the coronary tree. The increased temporal sampling (one temporal control point at every second projection image for the employed 133 projections protocol) is more robust against heart rate variations and fast movement.

2.4 Evaluation

During the development of a new reconstruction algorithm, the question whether one reconstructed image is better than another one needs to be answered. Also, different algorithms should be compared with respect to their result quality. Therefore, different methods can be found in the literature to evaluate the results of algorithms for the motion-compensated reconstruction of coronary arteries.

One easily accessible method is of course the qualitative evaluation of results by one or more human observers. Ratings can be captured, for example, with a 5-point Likert scale [Like 32], allowing for a statistical analysis of the results. Although it is an important part of any evaluation, since the subjective quality impression must be taken into account, it lacks the reproducibility and quantitative evidence of physical measurements.

Regarding quantitative evaluation of results, ground truth-based and ground truth-free methods can be differentiated. If a ground truth is available, an absolute statement about the achieved correctness of a reconstruction can be made. Unfortunately, this mostly limits experiments to phantom studies, as an exact ground truth from real human patient data is seldom available. Some studies performed an evaluation using a physical phantom [Mova 04, Jand 09b, Rohk 09b, Yang 09, Rohk 10b]. This takes all physical effects of the image acquisition into account and is therefore the most realistic phantom study. On the other hand, creation of the phantom and measurement of the ground truth is laborious and expensive. Therefore, others have relied on software phantoms. [Lore 04] proposed to model the coronary artery tree as a mean model from a pool of clinical data. [Yang 12] built a software phantom from annotated CT data. A very comprehensive phantom-based evaluation framework is CAVAREV [Rohk 10c]. It is based on the XCAT phantom [Sega 99, Sega 08] and provides simulated X-ray projection data from a real C-arm geometry, including breathing motion, if desired. What makes CAVAREV stand out is that it also provides a public platform where the phantom data can be downloaded and reconstruction results submitted. The evaluation of the quality metrics is then performed by the online platform, allowing for a public comparison of different approaches. CAVAREV is introduced in more detail in Chapter 5.

A quantitative evaluation also needs a metric. When a ground truth is available, this metric compares different properties of the reconstruction with that ground truth. A simple metric is the (root-)mean-squared error of voxels [Schä 06, Hans 08a]. Directly comparing voxel values has the downside that a geometrically correct reconstruction can still score low if its intensity values are different to the ground truth. Therefore, geometric measurements like a radius error [Hans 08b, Rohk 10b] have also been used. If a binary ground truth is available, the Dice coefficient can be used to compare the thresholded reconstruction with the ground truth [Rohk 10c]. This takes out any influence of the image intensity values. If no ground truth is available at all, image artefacts can be estimated by image noise [Schw 13b]. Finally, the sharpness of the coronary arteries has become a popular metric in the literature, also beyond C-arm CT [Li 01, Schw 13b, Schw 14a, Addy 15, Taub 15].

2.5   Summary and Conclusions

In this chapter, the state of the art of coronary artery reconstruction from rotational angiography ("C-arm CT") was presented and discussed. As a first distinction, methods can be classified into model-based and tomographic reconstruction methods, depending on whether they result in a centreline and/or lumen model or a tomographic image. The model-based methods were among the first to be found in the literature and share several aspects. Most of them require some form of manual interaction or a highly robust automatic centreline extraction on the acquired projection data. The former is not a desirable feature for interventional settings, while the latter is an unsolved task as of today. Second, lumen estimation is often a second step for these algorithms, which generally only result in a 3-D centreline model. Still, model-based algorithms have attractive properties like their ability to work with less-calibrated systems and their need for much less projection images compared to tomographic methods.

Tomographic reconstruction approaches can be further divided into iterative and analytical methods. Iterative approaches formulate the reconstruction problem as an optimisation problem and integrate the motion estimation into that. They are faced with high computational demands and a certain methodological complexity. On the other hand, they allow for great freedom in modelling different aspects of the acquisition process and introduced some underlying ideas into the field that can also be found in the approaches employing analytical reconstruction. A hybrid approach, where an analytical reconstruction is combined with an iterative optimisation of the motion model would be an example.

If a periodic heart motion is assumed, a correlation of the ECG signal recorded during the acquisition to the projection images used for an analytic reconstruction allows for an ECG-gated reconstruction. Several shapes, sizes and positions of the gating window have been proposed. Still, the current consensus is that these gated reconstructions provide good initial estimates for further motion estimation, but do not satisfy image quality expectations raised by recent motion compensation approaches.

Motion estimation and compensation approaches can be classified by the dimensionality of their motion model. Although the choice of a 3-D motion model and 3-D motion estimation seems natural, this leads to a high-dimensional optimisation problem. In addition, 3-D–3-D registration-based approaches suffer from the lack of image quality in gated reconstructions for most cardiac phases. Therefore, the 3-D approaches found in the literature use either periodicity assumptions or strong regularisation. The NOPMEC algorithm is also a 3-D motion estimation algorithm, but approaches the computational complexity by a simple cost function and an integration of the motion estimation into the highly optimised analytic reconstruction algorithm. Similar to 3-D–3-D approaches, 2-D–3-D registration-based methods suffer from high computational complexity and an ill-conditioned optimisation problem. Some approaches make use of easily detectable markers in the projection images. If such markers are not present, a non-deformable motion model could be used to limit the complexity by reducing the generality of the motion model. Finally, 2-D motion estimation approaches work directly on the acquired projection data and are therefore limited by the lack of depth information in the estimated motion. On the other hand, there is evidence that this is not a severe limitation for coronary artery motion [Unbe 15] (see also Chapter 4). In addition, the reduced dimensionality of the optimisation problem makes these approaches very enticing. So far, the methods presented in the literature either need detectable markers in the input data or an explicit vessel segmentation. Therefore, the intent of this work was to research the possibilities of a 2-D motion estimation and compensation method that neither requires markers nor an explicit vessel segmentation step.

2-D–2-D Motion Estimation and Compensation

In this chapter, a projection-based method for motion estimation and compensation is presented. We estimate motion by a deformable, multi-resolution, 2-D–2-D registration in projection space without requiring complex pre-processing steps like vessel centreline segmentation. The method is fully automatic, no user interaction is required.

As discussed in Chapter 2, cardiac C-arm CT is currently limited by the low temporal resolution of a straight-forward 3-D reconstruction. A retrospectively ECG-gated reconstruction of the X-ray projection data improves temporal resolution: Only images from a specific heart phase contribute to the reconstruction [Desj 04]. However, this presents a trade-off regarding the gating window size. Projection images within a small gating window are expected to display a similar motion state. But the small amount of data in turn leads to undersampling artefacts that strongly decrease 3-D image quality. On the other hand, a large gating window avoids undersampling artefacts, but then residual motion within the gated projection data again leads to motion artefacts.

The algorithm presented in this chapter uses an initial, ECG-gated reconstruction as a reference template for motion estimation. Since this image needs to show as little motion-related artefacts as possible to allow for a stable motion estimation, a smaller gating window is preferred initially. The resulting undersampling artefacts can be reduced by using a smooth ramp filter kernel, which unfortunately also reduces spatial resolution. Subsequent, motion-compensated reconstructions should be reconstructed from as many projection images as possible. This reduces the undersampling artefacts and allows the use of a sharper filter kernel. But motion estimation for projection images far from the reference heart phase (large gating window) is difficult without prior information. Therefore, we also show a method how motion estimation and compensation can be used to "bootstrap" a reconstruction with a large gating window and a sharper kernel in an iterative manner.

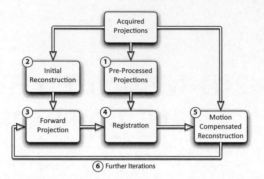

Figure 3.1: Illustration of the proposed algorithm.

In Section 3.1, the algorithm and all of its components are presented. This is followed by a complexity analysis in Section 3.2. Since most algorithm parameters are kept fixed in all following chapters, they are discussed in Section 3.3. Section 3.4 summarises this chapter.

Parts of this chapter have been published in [Schw 12, Schw 13b, Schw 13a].

3.1   Algorithm

The outline of our algorithm, which is also the outline of this section, is given by Figure 3.1 and Algorithm 3.1. In step 1, a copy of the original projection images is pre-processed using a morphological top-hat filter and a thresholding operation to reduce background structures. In step 2, an initial ECG-gated reconstruction is performed. In step 3, a thresholding operation removes non-vascular structures from the volume. In the same step, this sparse volume is then forward projected using the acquisition geometry. In these forward projection images (FwP), the region of interest, i.e. the region containing the contrasted vascular structure, is determined automatically. In step 4, the forward projections are registered to the pre-processed original projection images using deformable 2-D–2-D registration in a multi-resolution scheme. In step 5, a motion-compensated, ECG-gated reconstruction is performed using the deformation field from the registration step. In step 6, the procedure may be repeated for additional refinement using the same or different parameters.

3.1.1   Pre-Processing of Original Projections

Since the contrasted vessels are small objects with a larger-scale background, a background reduction of the original projection images $p(i, \boldsymbol{u})$ improves vessel contrast and increases stability of the registration process (i is the number of the image and $\boldsymbol{u}$ the pixel position). We use a morphological top-hat filter [Hans 08a] for this step. The filter has a circular structuring element of radius $r_{\mathrm{se,th}}$. Let $\mathcal{N}_{r_{\mathrm{se,th}}}(\boldsymbol{u})$ be the

---

Algorithm 3.1: 2-D–2-D motion estimation and compensation.

Input: Acquired projection images $p\left(i, \boldsymbol{u}\right)$

Output: Motion-compensated reconstruction $f_{h_r, \hat{\mathrm{M}}}\left(\boldsymbol{x}\right)$ and motion model $\hat{\mathrm{M}}$

// Step 1: Pre-processing of original projections

1 **for** $i \leftarrow 1$ **to** N **do**

2 $\quad$ Compute $p_{\mathsf{th}}\left(i, \boldsymbol{u}\right)$ (Eq. 3.1)

3 $\quad$ Determine q_{t_p} as the t_p percentile value of the largest pixel values in $p_{\mathsf{th}}\left(i, \boldsymbol{u}\right)$

4 $\quad$ $p_{\mathsf{bgr}}\left(i, \boldsymbol{u}\right) \leftarrow \begin{cases} p_{\mathsf{th}}\left(i, \boldsymbol{u}\right) & , p_{\mathsf{th}}\left(i, \boldsymbol{u}\right) \geq q_{t_p} \\ 0 & , \text{otherwise} \end{cases}$

5 **end**

// Step 2: Initial reconstruction

6 Compute $\hat{f}_{h_r}\left(\boldsymbol{x}\right)$ (Eq. 3.5)

7 **for** iter $\leftarrow 1$ **to** N_{iter} **do**

$\quad$ // Step 3: Forward projection generation

8 $\quad$ Determine q_{t_r} as the t_r percentile value of the largest voxel values in $\hat{f}_{h_r}\left(\boldsymbol{x}\right)$

9 $\quad$ $\hat{f}'_{h_r}\left(\boldsymbol{x}\right) \leftarrow \begin{cases} \hat{f}_{h_r}\left(\boldsymbol{x}\right) & , q_{t_r} \leq \hat{f}_{h_r}\left(\boldsymbol{x}\right) \leq q_{t_r} + W_r \\ 0 & , \text{otherwise} \end{cases}$

10 $\quad$ **foreach** $i \in \{1, \ldots, N\}$ **where** $\lambda\left(i, h_r\right) > 0$ **do**

11 $\quad\quad$ Compute $p_{\mathsf{fwp}}\left(i, \boldsymbol{u}\right)$ (Eq. 3.6)

12 $\quad$ **end**

13 $\quad$ Compute ROI (Alg. 3.2)

$\quad$ // Step 4: Image registration

14 $\quad$ **foreach** $i \in \{1, \ldots, N\}$ **where** $\lambda\left(i, h_r\right) > 0$ **do**

15 $\quad\quad$ $\hat{\mathrm{M}}\left(i, \cdot\right) \leftarrow \mathrm{argmin}_{\mathrm{M}(i, \cdot)} -\mathrm{NCC}_i\left(p_{\mathsf{bgr}}, p_{\mathsf{fwp}}, \mathrm{M}\right)$

16 $\quad$ **end**

$\quad$ // Step 5: Motion-compensated reconstruction

17 $\quad$ Compute $f_{h_r, \hat{\mathrm{M}}}\left(\boldsymbol{x}\right)$ (Eq. 3.11)

18 $\quad$ **if** iter $< N_{\mathsf{iter}}$ **then**

19 $\quad\quad$ $\hat{f}_{h_r}\left(\boldsymbol{x}\right) \leftarrow f_{h_r, \hat{\mathrm{M}}}\left(\boldsymbol{x}\right)$

20 $\quad$ **end**

21 **end**

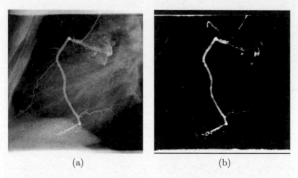

(a)   (b)

Figure 3.2: Original (left) and pre-processed (right) projection image. Images were cropped to the detected ROI for better visualisation.

neighbourhood around pixel position $\boldsymbol{u}$ defined by the structuring element. Then the top-hat filtered image is given by

$$p_{\text{th}}\left(i, \boldsymbol{u}\right) \;=\; p\left(i, \boldsymbol{u}\right) - \max_{\boldsymbol{u}' \in \mathcal{N}_{r_{\text{se,th}}}(\boldsymbol{u})} \tilde{p}_{\text{th}}\left(i, \boldsymbol{u}'\right) \text{ and} \tag{3.1}$$

$$\tilde{p}_{\text{th}}\left(i, \boldsymbol{u}\right) \;=\; \min_{\boldsymbol{u}'' \in \mathcal{N}_{r_{\text{se,th}}}(\boldsymbol{u})} p\left(i, \boldsymbol{u}''\right) \;. \tag{3.2}$$

This means that morphological opening (erosion followed by dilation) is performed and the result is subtracted from the original image. The effect of this operation is that all image structures larger than the structuring element are removed.

After filtering, a thresholding operation retains only the $t_p \in [0, 1]$ percentile of the largest pixel values. After both steps, most of the non-vascular background is removed (cf. Figure 3.2) and we denote the pre-processed projection images with $p_{\text{bgr}}\left(i, \boldsymbol{u}\right)$.

3.1.2   Initial Reconstruction

We perform an initial, ECG-gated reconstruction by inserting a weighting function λ into a standard FDK-type algorithm [Schä 06, Rohk 08b]. Let $h_r \in [0, 1]$ be the reference heart phase, at which reconstruction shall be carried out. The ECG-gated FDK reconstruction $f_{h_r} : \mathbb{R}^3 \mapsto \mathbb{R}$ at a voxel $\boldsymbol{x} \in \mathbb{R}^3$ is given by

$$f_{h_r}\left(\boldsymbol{x}\right) = \sum_{i=1}^{N} \lambda\left(i, h_r\right) \cdot w\left(i, \boldsymbol{x}\right) \cdot p_{\text{F}}\left(i, \text{A}\left(i, \boldsymbol{x}\right)\right) \;, \tag{3.3}$$

where N is the number of projection images, $w : \mathbb{N} \times \mathbb{R}^3 \mapsto \mathbb{R}$ is the FDK distance weight and $p_{\text{F}}\left(i, \boldsymbol{u}\right) : \mathbb{N} \times \mathbb{R}^2 \mapsto \mathbb{R}$ is the filtered, redundancy- and cosine-weighted projection data of the i-th image at pixel position $\boldsymbol{u}$. The pixel position for backprojection to the voxel $\boldsymbol{x}$ is determined by the perspective projection

$A : \mathbb{N} \times \mathbb{R}^3 \mapsto \mathbb{R}^2, (i, \boldsymbol{x}) \mapsto A(i, \boldsymbol{x}) = \boldsymbol{u}$. The perspective projection A can be calculated using pre-calibrated projection matrices [Wies 00]. The ECG-gating weighting function λ used here is a cosine window introduced in [Rohk 08b]:

$$\lambda(l, h_r) = \begin{cases} \cos^a\left(\frac{d(h(i), h_r)}{\omega}\pi\right) & , d(h(i), h_i) \leq \frac{\omega}{2} \\ 0 & , \text{ otherwise} \end{cases}, \qquad (3.4)$$

where $h(i)$ is the heart phase of the i-th projection image according to the ECG, $\omega \in [0, 1]$ controls the width and $a \geq 0$ controls the shape of the gating window. The distance measure d is defined as $d(h_1, h_2) = \min_{j \in \{0,1,-1\}} |h_1 - h_2 + j|$.

Since the resulting reconstruction suffers from undersampling artefacts, we also perform a streak reduction. A formal derivation of this post-processing step was presented in [Rohk 08b]. In practice, streak reduction is integrated into the reconstruction as follows:

$$\hat{f}_{h_r}(\boldsymbol{x}) = \sum_{i=1+N_{\text{ign}}}^{N-N_{\text{ign}}} \lambda(j_i, h_r) \cdot w(j_i, \boldsymbol{x}) \cdot p_{\text{F}}(j_i, A(j_i, \boldsymbol{x})) \quad , \qquad (3.5)$$

with an enforced ordering of $\lambda(j_1, h_r) \cdot w(j_1, \boldsymbol{x}) \cdot p_{\text{F}}(j_1, A(j_i, \boldsymbol{x})) \leq \cdots \leq \lambda(j_N, h_r) \cdot w(j_N, \boldsymbol{x}) \cdot p_{\text{F}}(j_N, A(j_N, \boldsymbol{x}))$ and $j_i \in \{1, \dots, N\}$, $N_{\text{ign}} \in \mathbb{N}_0$. This means the N_{ign} smallest and largest contributions to each voxel are ignored during reconstruction. Voxel-driven backprojection is done on graphics hardware [Hofm 11].

3.1.3   Forward Projection Generation

Thresholding

Only contrasted vascular structure is of interest for the registration algorithm, which means only high-contrast structure needs to be retained. Since a selective contrasting is performed during the acquisition, vascular structure is the predominant high-contrast structure in the image. Therefore, a simple thresholding operation can be employed to remove background structures: Only the $t_r \in [0, 1]$ percentile of the largest voxel values is retained, while the other voxels are set to 0. Additionally, all voxel values larger than the t_r percentile plus a grey value window of size W_r are also set to 0 to limit the influence of artefacts. We denote the thresholded initial reconstruction with $\hat{f}'_{h_r}(\boldsymbol{x})$.

Forward Projection

After the thresholding of the initial reconstruction, maximum intensity forward projection images $p_{\text{fwp}}(i, \boldsymbol{u}) : \mathbb{N} \times \mathbb{R}^2 \mapsto \mathbb{R}$ are generated using the original acquisition geometry. Only those projections with a gating weight $\lambda(i, h_r) > 0$ need to be generated, since others will not be used by the motion-compensated reconstruction. We use a ray-casting approach as in [Gali 03]:

$$p_{\text{fwp}}(i, \boldsymbol{u}) = \max_{\boldsymbol{x} \in L_{i,\boldsymbol{u}}} \hat{f}'_{h_r}(\boldsymbol{x}) \quad , \qquad (3.6)$$

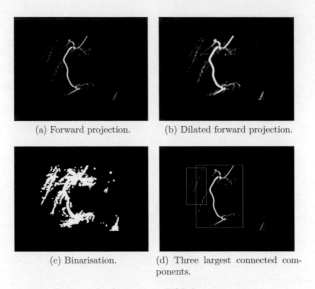

(a) Forward projection.   (b) Dilated forward projection.

(c) Binarisation.   (d) Three largest connected com-
                                ponents.

Figure 3.3: Automatic ROI determination.

where $L_{i,u} = \{x \in \mathbb{R}^3 \mid \mathrm{A}(i, x) = u\}$ is the set of voxels representing the virtual X-ray beam from the i-th source position to pixel position u on the detector (pixel-driven ray-casting). Forward projections are generated in parallel on graphics hardware [Wein 08]. No consideration of ray intersection length is necessary due to the maximum intensity projection mode.

Region of Interest Detection

The registration process can be sped up and stabilised by defining a region of interest (ROI) for the evaluation of the objective function. This ROI is automatically determined from the forward projections by applying Algorithm 3.2 to every forward-projected image (cf. Figure 3.3):

First, the forward projection image is dilated with a circular structuring element to close small gaps between vessel segments that might have been created by the thresholding. Then the image is binarised and connected components are labelled. With the assumption that the coronary tree is the largest connected component, the bounding box of this component is returned for this image.

The final ROI is the bounding box covering the bounding boxes from all projection images, with an added safety margin to account for incomplete structure in the initial reconstruction. Algorithm 3.2 can be executed in parallel for all forward projections, only the final ROI calculation needs to be done after all individual bounding boxes are found.

Algorithm 3.2: Region of interest detection.

Input: Forward-projected image $p_{\mathsf{fwp}}(i, \boldsymbol{u})$
Output: Region of interest ROI

   /* Dilate $p_{\mathsf{fwp}}(i, \boldsymbol{u})$ using morphological operations [Doug 03] with a
      circular structuring element of radius $r_{\mathsf{se,roi}}$.   */
1 $p_{\mathsf{fwp,dil}}(i, \boldsymbol{u}) \leftarrow$ dilate$(p_{\mathsf{fwp}}(i, \boldsymbol{u}), r_{\mathsf{se,roi}})$

   // Binarise the image.

2 $p_{\mathsf{fwp,bin}}(i, \boldsymbol{u}) \leftarrow \begin{cases} 1 & , \, p_{\mathsf{fwp,dil}}(i, \boldsymbol{u}) > 0 \\ 0 & , \, \text{otherwise} \end{cases}$

   /* Detect and label connected components [Shap 00, Chapter 3, pp.
      503-506], compute component sizes as the number of pixels in
      each component.   */
3 cc $\leftarrow$ connectedComponents$(p_{\mathsf{fwp,bin}}(i, \boldsymbol{u}))$

   // Find the largest object.

4 $l \leftarrow$ argmax$_i$ size(cc[i])

   // Calculate its rectangular bounding box.

5 **return** ROI $\leftarrow$ boundingBox(cc[l])

3.1.4   Image Registration

During image registration, a mapping between the space of the pre-processed projection images $p_{\mathsf{bgr}}(i, \boldsymbol{u})$ and the forward projections $p_{\mathsf{fwp}}(i, \boldsymbol{u})$ is established. After registration, $p_{\mathsf{bgr}}(i, \mathrm{M}(i, \boldsymbol{u}))$ is similar to $p_{\mathsf{fwp}}(i, \boldsymbol{u})$, where $\mathrm{M} : \mathbb{N} \times \mathbb{R}^2 \mapsto \mathbb{R}^2, \mathrm{M}(i, \boldsymbol{u}) = \boldsymbol{u}'$ is the motion vector field for the i-th image. Similarity is defined by the objective function of the registration algorithm.

    The registration framework is built using the Insight Segmentation and Registration Toolkit (ITK)[1].

Motion Model

We employ a multi-resolution scheme with an affine motion model on all resolution levels, and an additional uniform cubic B-spline motion model on the higher levels:

$$\mathrm{M}(i, \boldsymbol{u}) = \mathrm{M}_{\mathsf{affine}}(i, \boldsymbol{u}) + \mathrm{M}_{\mathsf{spline}}(i, \boldsymbol{u}) \quad . \tag{3.7}$$

    This separation of affine and deformable motion as well as the multi-resolution scheme reduce the susceptibility of the deformable registration to local minima and also increase convergence speed.

    The affine motion model

$$\mathrm{M}_{\mathsf{affine}}(i, \boldsymbol{u}) = \boldsymbol{A}_i \cdot \boldsymbol{u} + \boldsymbol{t}_i \quad , \tag{3.8}$$

with linear transformation $\boldsymbol{A}_i \in \mathbb{R}^{2 \times 2}$ and translation vector $\boldsymbol{t}_i \in \mathbb{R}^2$, has 6 degrees of freedom per image, representing anisotropic scaling, shear, rotation and translation.

---

[1]http://www.itk.org/

Note that the affine parameters are only estimated on those resolution levels where no deformable component is present. When the B-spline motion model is added, the last affine parameters are kept fixed and only the deformable component's parameters are estimated.

The B-spline motion model

$$\mathrm{M}_{\mathrm{spline}}\left(i, \boldsymbol{u}\right) = \boldsymbol{u} + \sum_{j=1}^{c^2} \beta\left(|u_x - k_{j,x}|\right) \cdot \beta\left(|u_y - k_{j,y}|\right) \cdot \boldsymbol{s}_{i,j} \tag{3.9}$$

is parameterised by the number of control points c in each dimension, resulting in $2 \cdot c^2$ degrees of freedom per image. $\boldsymbol{k}_j \in \mathbb{R}^2$ are the control point locations, $\boldsymbol{s}_{i,j} \in \mathbb{R}^2$ the B-spline coefficient vectors and $\beta\left(x\right) : \mathbb{R} \mapsto \mathbb{R}$ are the B-spline basis functions [Unse 99].

The choice of c influences the relation of smoothness (small c) to flexibility (large c) of the motion model. It is important to note that the motion model is always defined on the whole image region. The ROI is only used for the evaluation of the objective function.

Multi-Resolution Scheme

When performing registration with a parametric motion model (i.e. B-splines) and a multi-resolution scheme, there exist two possibilities of realising the multi-resolution behaviour. First, the motion model(s) can be defined in physical coordinates with fixed parameters and the images are rescaled. The motion models are therefore independent of the current pixel size of a scaled projection image. When the pixel resolution is decreased, small-scale structures vanish and registration focuses on the larger structures. This leads to a registration process that performs a coarser alignment first, with increasing refinement of smaller structures as resolution increases.

The second possibility is leaving the projection images as-is and instead changing the parameters of the motion model(s). This has essentially the same effect, although the impact of a parameter change is not as intuitive as a rescaling of the images.

We used a combination of both approaches: For "easier" registration tasks with small gating window sizes, motion model parameters are kept fixed and only the image size and resolution are changed. For the more difficult problem of large ω, the flexibility of the B-spline motion model is increased together with the image resolution. In the remainder of this chapter, we denote the number of resolution levels with R.

Objective Function

We use normalised cross-correlation (NCC) as the similarity measure, which is a common measure for multi-modality registration problems [Russ 03]. Purely intensity-based metrics like sum of squared differences do not work for this problem, since the grey values of $p_{\mathrm{bgr}}\left(i, \boldsymbol{u}\right)$ and $p_{\mathrm{fwp}}\left(i, \boldsymbol{u}\right)$ differ due to the gated reconstruction and the maximum intensity forward projection. NCC is insensitive to these grey value differences, while being parameter-free and less computationally intensive than mutual information or similar multi-modality metrics. The NCC is only evaluated within the

Algorithm 3.3: *RegularStepGradientDescentOptimizer* from ITK. Shown for optimisation of B-spline model parameters.

Input: Initial parameter set s, maxSteps, minGrad, Initial stepLength, relaxFac, minStepLength
Output: Final parameter set $\hat{s}$

1 curStep $\leftarrow 0$
2 $\hat{s} \leftarrow s$
3 **while true do**
  // Maximum number of steps reached?
4   **if** curStep $\geq$ maxSteps **then break**
  // Calculate gradient of objective function
5   $\Delta s \leftarrow -\nabla \text{NCC}_i \left(p_{\text{bgr}}, p_{\text{fwp}}, \text{M} \right)$
  // Minimum gradient reached?
6   **if** $\|\Delta s\| <$ minGrad **then break**
  // Change of direction, i.e. overshoot?
7   **if** $\Delta s^{(curStep-1)} \cdot \Delta s^T < 0$ **then**
8   │   stepLength $\leftarrow$ stepLength $\cdot$ relaxFac
9   **end**
  // Minimum step length reached?
10   **if** stepLength $<$ minStepLength **then break**
11   fac $\leftarrow -$stepLength $/ \|\Delta s\|$
12   $\hat{s} \leftarrow \hat{s} +$ fac $\cdot \Delta s$
13 **end**

ROI, which also decreases computation time. NCC for projection image i is defined as

$$\text{NCC}_i\left(p_{\text{bgr}}, p_{\text{fwp}}, \text{M}\right) = \frac{1}{n-1} \left\langle \frac{\boldsymbol{P}_{i,\text{bgr}}}{\|\boldsymbol{P}_{i,\text{bgr}}\|}, \frac{\boldsymbol{P}_{i,\text{fwp}}}{\|\boldsymbol{P}_{i,\text{fwp}}\|} \right\rangle \ , \qquad (3.10)$$

where n is the number of pixels in the ROI, $\langle \star, \star \rangle$ is the inner product and $\|\star\|$ the L^2 norm. $\boldsymbol{P}_{i,\text{bgr}}\left(\boldsymbol{u}\right) = p_{\text{bgr}}\left(i, \text{M}\left(i, \boldsymbol{u}\right)\right) - \overline{p_{\text{bgr}}}\left(i\right)$ and $\boldsymbol{P}_{i,\text{fwp}}\left(\boldsymbol{u}\right) = p_{\text{fwp}}\left(i, \boldsymbol{u}\right) - \overline{p_{\text{fwp}}}\left(i\right)$, where $\overline{p_{\star}}\left(i\right)$ is the mean intensity of an image. The transformed images $p_{\text{bgr}}\left(i, \text{M}\left(i, \boldsymbol{u}\right)\right)$ need only be computed at those pixels necessary for the evaluation of the NCC, i.e. within the ROI. Bilinear interpolation is used as image transformation. The calculation of the NCC can be sped up by caching the B-spline weights for all pixels, since the ROI and B-spline grid points do not change during registration. The faster implementation is available online[2].

Registration is driven by a gradient descent optimisation method. The *RegularStepGradientDescentOptimizer* of ITK is used, which does not do a line search, but scales the step size with relaxFac if the direction of the gradient changes (cf. Algorithm 3.3). This can lead to oscillation, since one optimisation step is not guaranteed to decrease the objective function value in every case. On the other hand, no overhead by a line search is induced.

Since we perform registration on a per-image basis, all projections can be processed in parallel.

3.1.5 Motion-Compensated Reconstruction

After registration, the motion vector field $\text{M}\left(i, \boldsymbol{u}\right)$ is known for every projection image. The estimated motion can be compensated for in the backprojection step (cf. Figure 3.4)

$$f_{h_r,\text{M}}\left(\boldsymbol{x}\right) = \sum_{i=1}^{N} \lambda\left(i, h_r\right) \cdot w\left(i, \boldsymbol{x}\right) \cdot p_{\text{F}}\left(i, \text{M}\left(i, \text{A}\left(i, \boldsymbol{x}\right)\right)\right) \ . \qquad (3.11)$$

The benefit of this approach is that the application of the motion model is a simple coordinate transform. The only interpolation of pixel values happens during the evaluation of $p_{\text{F}}\left(i, \boldsymbol{u}'\right)$, which is necessary in any case. Another approach, which was used in previous work on projection-based motion estimation, would be to deform the projection images and perform a normal backprojection. But this introduces an additional interpolation of pixel values in the projection domain. Of course, the distance weight $w\left(i, \boldsymbol{x}\right)$ is incorrect in Equation 3.11, since it belongs to the original detector location $\boldsymbol{u}$. In the same way, the filtered pixel value at position $\boldsymbol{u}'$ is incorrect. The ramp filter kernel for filtered backprojection is designed for static reconstruction. When motion is introduced, the desired cancellation effects for contributions from different angulations do not work as expected anymore. Therefore, $f_{h_r,\text{M}}\left(\boldsymbol{x}\right)$ is only an approximate solution. But the influence of these issues is only negligible (especially for high-contrast imaging), as demonstrated by the good experiences with a similar reconstruction method for 3-D motion in previous work [Schä 06, Camm 10, Rohk 10b, Mull 13].

---

[2]http://www5.cs.fau.de/our-team/schwemmer-chris/software/

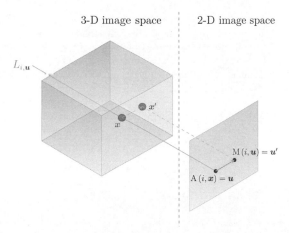

Figure 3.4: Illustration of the motion-compensated backprojection process with a 2-D motion vector field. For a given projection image i and voxel $\boldsymbol{x}$, the detector position $\boldsymbol{u}$ is given by the perspective projection function $A(i, \boldsymbol{x}) = \boldsymbol{u}$. The structure located at $\boldsymbol{x}$ when at the reference heart phase h_r moves to $\boldsymbol{x}'$ at time point i. The corresponding detector position is given by $M(i, \boldsymbol{u}) = \boldsymbol{u}'$. The pixel value at $\boldsymbol{u}'$ is then backprojected to the original voxel position $\boldsymbol{x}$.

Backprojection can be implemented very efficiently on graphics hardware [Hofm 11]. The B-spline weights can again be pre-calculated and then cached in the texture unit of the graphics card together with the current set of coefficients $\{\boldsymbol{s}_{i,\cdot}\}$. Therefore, the motion-compensated backprojection can be carried out completely parallelised on the graphics card.

The same streak reduction as in Equation 3.5 is also used for the motion-compensated reconstruction when less than 100 % of the projection data are used. For the sake of conciseness, this is not shown in Equation 3.11, since the streak reduction is not the focus here.

3.1.6   Further Iterations

The motion compensation algorithm can be used in an iterative manner: The output from step 3.1.5 can be used as input for step 3.1.3. Registration accuracy with the same set of parameters may improve when using input images that contain less artefacts and better contrast than the initial reconstruction. In addition to that, the parameters can also be changed between iterations. This allows a successive increase in gating window size and flexibility of the motion model, or a different ramp filter kernel (with better spatial resolution) for the motion-compensated reconstruction.

Since the initial reconstruction must be performed without any motion compensation, a small gating window is needed to avoid residual motion as much as possible. Still, remaining motion inside that window degrades image quality, which can be compensated by the algorithm described in this chapter. A direct increase of ω in the first iteration is difficult for two reasons: Both residual motion and undersampling artefacts from the small window size limit the quality of the reference image, increasing the chance of misregistration during motion estimation. We therefore increase ω in an iterative fashion. For a certain ω, residual motion is compensated and the result used as a reference image for a new iteration with increased ω and c.

Besides a better reference image, a new iteration can also use the estimated motion vector field from the previous iteration as prior knowledge. This can help to speed up and stabilise the motion estimation process. Note that, if ω is increased, only motion models for projection images within the previous, smaller gating window are available, of course.

3.2 Complexity Analysis

For this analysis, we assume the side length of the projection images and the side length of reconstructed volumes to be of the same order of magnitude. Let n therefore denote either.

The pre-processing step needs to go through all pixels of all projections images three times (top-hat filtering, percentile determination and thresholding), resulting in a time complexity of

$$\mathcal{O}\left(Nn^2\right) . \tag{3.12}$$

Backprojection for the initial reconstruction has a time complexity of

$$\mathcal{O}\left(Nn^3\right) , \tag{3.13}$$

since every voxel needs to be accessed for every projection image.

The forward projection step consists of three parts. First, the threshold is calculated and applied, which has a time complexity of $\mathcal{O}\left(n^3\right)$. Then, the actual forward projection is calculated, which casts a ray from every pixel of every projection image through the volume, resulting in a time complexity of $\mathcal{O}\left(Nn^3\right)$. Third, automatic ROI determination accesses all pixels of all projection images multiple times, i.e. $\mathcal{O}\left(Nn^2\right)$. Therefore, the total time complexity of this step is

$$\mathcal{O}\left(Nn^3\right) . \tag{3.14}$$

The registration step consists of several loops: For every projection image, every resolution level and every optimisation step, every pixel needs to be accessed for the calculation of the objective function (since the ROI could be the whole image in the worst case). With R being the number of resolution levels, let k be the maximum number of optimisation steps allowed. Then the time complexity of the registration algorithm without motion model evaluation is

$$\mathcal{O}\left(NRkn^2\right) . \tag{3.15}$$

Strictly speaking, the calculation of the gradient of the objective function has an additional time complexity of $\mathcal{O}\left(c^2\right)$: It needs to update every coefficient of the

B-spline field. But this can be neglected in 3.15, since clearly $n \gg c$. The same holds for the affine part.

Since B-splines have a locality property, i.e. evaluation at a specific point only depends on a local neighbourhood, the time complexity of B-spline evaluation does not depend on c and can therefore be neglected in terms of the $\mathcal{O}$ calculus. The same argument can be used for the time complexity of motion-compensated backprojection, which is therefore equivalent to 3.13.

The time complexity of one complete iteration of the whole algorithm depends on whether $Rk > n$ and therefore $\mathcal{O}(NRkn^2) > \mathcal{O}(Nn^3)$ or vice versa. For practical purposes, the difference is small, because with the parameters presented in the next section, actually $Rk \approx n$ and therefore the final time complexity can be estimated to be within

$$\mathcal{O}\left(Nn^3\right) . \tag{3.16}$$

Of course, all observations consider a straight-forward implementation and no parallelisation effects, since this is not reflected by the $\mathcal{O}$-calculus. But in practice, back- and forward projection can be parallelised over all n^3 voxels and n^2 pixels, while registration can only be parallelised over all N projection images.

3.3   Parameter Settings

Pre-processing of the projection images is performed using $r_{\mathrm{se,th}} = 3.85\,\mathrm{mm}$ and $t_p = 0.2$. The initial reconstruction is generated with a gating window of size $\omega = 0.4$, shape parameter $a = 4$ and $N_{\mathrm{ign}} = 3$ together with a smooth filter kernel. Before forward projection, volumetric images are processed with $t_r = 0.005$ and $W_r = 1600\,\mathrm{GV}$. Due to the ECG gating, intermediate volumes are not scaled to Hounsfield units, which is why W_r is given in GV (grey values). The region of interest detection uses $r_{\mathrm{se,roi}} = 1.54\,\mathrm{mm}$ (5 pixels) and a safety margin of $\approx 3\,\mathrm{mm}$ (10 pixels).

In total, $N_{\mathrm{iter}} = 3$ algorithm iterations are performed. For iterations 1 and 2, the parameters of the initial reconstruction ($\omega = 0.4$, $a = 4$, $N_{\mathrm{ign}} = 3$, smooth filter kernel) are used for motion-compensated reconstruction. In iteration 3, the gating window size is increased to either $\omega = 0.8$, $a = 4$ with $N_{\mathrm{ign}} = 3$, or to $\omega = 1.0$, $a = 0$ with $N_{\mathrm{ign}} = 0$. The latter corresponds to a non-gated reconstruction using all projection data. For iteration 3, a normal filter kernel is used.

For iterations 1 and 2, the multi-resolution scheme and motion model configuration shown in Figure 3.5a is used. It has three resolution levels. On the lower two, $\mathrm{M_{affine}}(i, \boldsymbol{u})$ is estimated. Only on the highest level (original projection image resolution), $\mathrm{M_{spline}}(i, \boldsymbol{u})$ with $c = 6$ is estimated.

For iteration 3 the configuration shown in Figure 3.5b is employed. It has five resolution levels. Only on the lowest level, $\mathrm{M_{affine}}(i, \boldsymbol{u})$ is estimated. On levels 2 and 3, $\mathrm{M_{spline}}(i, \boldsymbol{u})$ with $c = 6$ and on levels 4 and 5, $\mathrm{M_{spline}}(i, \boldsymbol{u})$ with $c = 12$ is estimated.

The resize factor between the different resolution levels is always 2. Downscaling of the images between resolution levels is performed by bilinear interpolation and pre-smoothing with a Gaussian kernel ($\sigma = 1$). Optimisation on one resolution level is stopped after reaching maxSteps = 200 (affine motion model) or maxSteps = 250 (B-spline motion model). Additionally, optimisation is stopped if the gradient magnitude

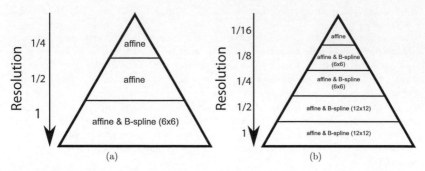

Figure 3.5: Multi-resolution schemes employed. (a) Scheme used for $\omega = 0.4$ with 3 resolution levels and $\mathrm{M_{spline}}\,(i, \boldsymbol{u})$ only on the highest level. (b) Scheme used for $\omega \geq 0.8$ with 5 resolution levels and two different c.

of the NCC is below minGrad $= 1 \cdot 10^{-7}$ (affine motion model) or minGrad $= 3 \cdot 10^{-4}$ (B-spline motion model). Since the numerical scales of the elements of $\boldsymbol{A}_i$ and $\boldsymbol{t}_i$ are vastly different, the gradient components of $\boldsymbol{t}_i$ are scaled by $1 \cdot 10^{-7}$ before computing the step length of the gradient descent optimiser. The initial step length is stepLength $= 16$, the minimum step length is minStepLength $= 0.01$, with relaxFac $= 0.7$.

Iteration 2 does not use the motion model from iteration 1 as previous knowledge, whereas in iteration 3, the previous motion model is used as a starting point for all projections where it is available. In the 5-level scheme of this iteration, the previous motion model (which has $c = 6$) is used as input to the $1/2$ resolution level while skipping lower levels. That means that for projections with previous knowledge available, only registration on the two highest resolution levels is performed instead of on all five.

The choice of gating and registration parameters comes from the following rationale: The initial reconstruction is assumed to be of bad quality. Therefore, a second iteration with the same parameters is performed to enhance registration accuracy. Then the gating window size is increased in the third iteration. This demands a more flexible motion model ($c = 12$ instead of 6), which in turn makes a more elaborate multi-resolution scheme necessary. A larger ω decreases undersampling artefacts and allows the use of a sharper ramp filter kernel, which in turn increases spatial resolution.

It should be noted that the parameter settings presented here haven been optimised with regard to the protocol established in Section 1.3. Especially the image-dependent parameters such as structuring element sizes, thresholds and N_{ign} depend on the number of projection images acquired, their size and resolution, and the selected kV level.

3.4   Summary

In this chapter, a method for projection-based 2-D–2-D motion estimation using image registration was presented. It is embedded in an iterative algorithm for motion estimation and compensation. This algorithm does not require any complex segmentation or user interaction and is thus fully automatic. Before the first iteration, the algorithm is initialised with an ECG-gated reconstruction. The gating window size is a trade-off between undersampling and motion-related artefacts. The latter can be reduced by residual motion compensation. But motion estimation and compensation becomes more difficult with large window sizes. This can be overcome by the iterative algorithm that successively increases the window size in a bootstrapping process. The registration process is stabilised and sped up by a multi-resolution scheme that is adapted to the current flexibility of the motion model.

Henceforth, the presented algorithm shall be referenced as RMC (Registration-based Motion Compensation). In the following four chapters, RMC is evaluated first on a simple mathematical phantom, then using the CAVAREV platform, and finally in a large human clinical study.

Numerical Phantom Study

In this chapter, the RMC algorithm presented in Chapter 3.1 and the state-of-the-art algorithm NOPMEC are evaluated in a simulation study using a numerical phantom. The purpose of this study is to gain insight into the shape-preserving properties of the algorithms, as well as the dependence of the estimated motion vector field on the observed object itself. In addition, a study in a well-controlled and fully known environment allows using known-reference metrics that are not available in more complex setups. Since the algorithms are also evaluated on static datasets without any motion, an approximation of their inherent error can be established. The experimental setup is described in Section 4.1. The results of the study are presented in Section 4.2 and discussed in Section 4.3.

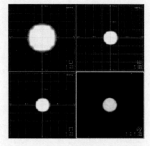 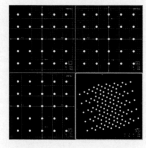

Figure 4.1: Implemented numerical phantoms reconstructed with a standard FDK-type algorithm. Left: Single sphere. Right: 5×5×5 sphere grid. Shown are a sagittal, coronal and axial plane through the middle of the phantom, as well as a 3-D rendering.

4.1   Experimental Setup

4.1.1   Numerical Phantom and Simulation Environment

The phantom used for this study consists of one or multiple spheres of homogeneous density in free space. The rationale behind using spheres is that errors during motion compensation directly map to a non-spherical result, allowing for a convenient qualitative visualisation. Quantitatively, shape measures for spheres are also easily calculated. Each sphere was of radius $r_{\text{sphere}} = 2\,\text{mm}$, which is in the normal size range of mid to distal main branches of coronary arteries [Dodg 92]. The spheres had the simulated material properties of iodine. Background density was set to 0, i.e. vacuum. Two instances of the phantom were generated. One contained a single sphere, the other a grid of 5×5×5 spheres (cf. Figure 4.1). The single sphere was placed 6 mm off-centre in x direction. The central sphere of the grid was also placed 6 mm off-centre in x direction. The grid was equally spaced in such a way that each sphere was exactly in the middle between neighbouring control points of the NOPMEC motion model (cf. Section 2.3). This resulted in a sphere-to-sphere distance of 24 mm.

The phantom was implemented inside the CONRAD software framework [Maie 13][1]. This allows for analytical projection image generation directly from the numerical phantom, without voxelisation [Maie 12]. In addition, this framework supports sophisticated time-based motion simulation. This was used here to generate a heart beat-like motion of the spheres. The concept implemented in CONRAD for this is that of time warping [Sega 01, Maie 13]. During simulation, a linear time $t \in [0, 1]$ is mapped to the generated projection images. Through time warping modules connected to each other, this linear mapping is transformed to a more complex relation. To generate a heart beat-like motion, the following time warping modules were used in succession:

1. Harmonic time warp: Resulting motion is a 5 times repetition of the original motion.

2. Rest phase of 20 %: Only in 80 % of the available time, motion occurs.

3. Periodic time warp: Resulting motion is a forward-backward cycle.

4. Sigmoid time warp: Resulting motion is an accelerated/decelerated motion.

The final resulting linear time – warped time relation is shown in Figure 4.2. This directly represents the motion the phantoms went through during simulation. Those projection images belonging to the 20 % rest phase were used to define the reference heart phase h_r for both motion estimation algorithms. The amplitude of the motion was set to 6 mm, its direction along the x axis.

Projection images were generated using a trajectory calibrated from a real Artis zee system (Siemens Healthcare GmbH, Forchheim, Germany), which represents a circular short scan trajectory with variances from an ideal circle due to mechanical inaccuracies. The system uses a flat panel detector with a size of $40 \times 30\,\text{cm}$ and an isotropic detector resolution of 0.308 mm. Source-detector-distance was ∼120 cm

---

[1]http://conrad.stanford.edu/

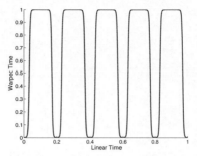

Figure 4.2: Linear time to warped time relationship.

with a source-isocentre-distance of ∼80 cm. 133 projection images with an angular spacing of 1.5° were generated for each simulation. Volumetric images were always reconstructed with a size of 256 × 256 × 196 voxels and an isotropic voxel size of 0.56 mm.

In total, four scenes were simulated and corresponding projection images created: A single sphere, both static and in motion. And the sphere grid, also both static and in motion. The resting position of an in-motion sphere corresponds to its position in the static scenes. From each of these datasets, seven reconstructions were generated:

1. Non-compensated, FDK-type reconstruction as a baseline (normal ramp filter kernel).

2. *Initial*: ECG-gated reconstruction without motion compensation ($\omega = 0.4$, $a = 4$, $N_{\mathrm{ign}} = 3$, smooth ramp filter kernel). This also serves as the reference volume for the NOPMEC algorithm.

3. RMC 40 %: Motion-compensated reconstruction with 2 iterations ($\omega = 0.4$, $a = 4$, $N_{\mathrm{ign}} = 3$, smooth ramp filter kernel).

4. RMC 80 %: Motion-compensated reconstruction with 3 iterations ($\omega = 0.8$, $a = 4$, $N_{\mathrm{ign}} = 3$, normal ramp filter kernel).

5. RMC 100 %: Motion-compensated reconstruction with 3 iterations ($\omega = 1.0$, $a = 0$, $N_{\mathrm{ign}} = 0$, normal ramp filter kernel).

6. NOPMEC: Motion-compensated reconstruction ($\omega - 1.0$, $a - 0$, $N_{\mathrm{ign}} - 0$, normal ramp filter kernel).

7. NOPMEC$_{\mathrm{limit}}$: Motion-compensated reconstruction ($\omega = 1.0$, $a = 0$, $N_{\mathrm{ign}} = 0$, normal ramp filter kernel) without motion in viewing direction.

The seventh reconstruction was generated by restricting the motion estimation of the NOPMEC algorithm to motion that is always perpendicular to the C-arm viewing direction at a given time point. In other words, the motion vector fields resulting from this do not contain depth information with respect to the corresponding viewing direction.

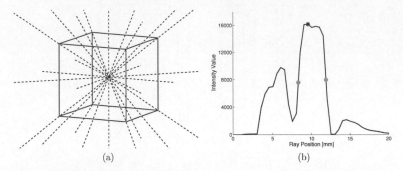

(a)   (b)

Figure 4.3: Shape measurement process. (a) Ray directions shown with the unit cube. (b) Diameter estimation on an intensity profile. Red star: Maximum. Green dots: Half-maximum. Distance between half-maxima is estimated diameter.

4.1.2 Metrics

Normalised cross-correlation (NCC) against the FDK reconstructions of the static datasets was used to assess all reconstructions. Comparison against FDK reconstructions instead of against a voxelised phantom was chosen to reduce the influence of the backprojection method itself on the metric.

Additionally, shape measures were calculated for the reconstructed spheres. From the ideal centre position of each sphere, 13 rays of length 20 mm were shot out and intensity profiles measured along the rays (using 10-fold subsampling). From the intensity profiles, full-width-at-half-maximum was used to estimate the diameter of the sphere along each ray. Figure 4.3 illustrates this process. In detail, the 13 ray directions used are the x, y and z axis, the four main diagonals connecting the corners of the unit cube, and the six diagonals halfway between two corners. Using the 13 diameter estimates per sphere, minimum and maximum as well as average and standard deviation were calculated. Assuming the reconstructed sphere to be an ellipsoid, the normalised linear eccentricity $e = \frac{\sqrt{a^2-b^2}}{r_{\text{sphere}}}$ was calculated. a and b are the semi-major and semi-minor axes of the ellipsoid, i.e. maximum/2 and minimum/2. The normalisation factor $r_{\text{sphere}} = 2\,\text{mm}$ is the radius of the phantom sphere to make e a dimension-less metric expressed in relation to the original sphere size. An ideal sphere has a linear eccentricity of 0.

For the sphere grid experiments, individual sphere measurements were grouped as follows: An overall summary over all $5 \times 5 \times 5$ spheres, the values of the centre sphere only, and the 98 outer spheres. For the summary and outer sphere statistics, minimum/maximum/mean diameter values in the tables were calculated over the spheres' mean diameters, not over all individual rays. The minimum/maximum/mean eccentricity values were calculated over the sphere's eccentricities.

Table 4.1: Normalised cross-correlation values against FDK reconstruction of static scene. Best values in each column are marked in bold.

	single, static	single, motion	grid, static	grid, motion
FDK	*1*	0.73	*1*	0.77
Initial	**0.93**	**0.93**	0.72	0.73
RMC 40%	0.75	0.75	0.72	0.72
RMC 80%	0.48	0.48	0.82	0.83
RMC 100%	0.51	0.51	**0.98**	**0.98**
NOPMEC	0.31	0.30	0.92	0.90
NOPMEC$_{limit}$	0.29	0.29	0.92	0.90

Table 4.2: Shape measures for single sphere experiments. Best values are marked in bold.

	Static Scene Diameter (mm)			e	Moving Scene Diameter (mm)			e
	min	max	mean		min	max	mean	
FDK	3.5	4.3	**3.6 ± 0.2**	0.650	3.5	3.5	**3.5 ± 0.0**	**0.177**
Initial	2.6	3.5	3.4 ± 0.3	**0.599**	2.6	3.5	3.4 ± 0.3	0.599
RMC 40%	4.2	5.2	4.7 ± 0.3	0.750	4.2	5.2	4.7 ± 0.3	0.750
RMC 80%	5.5	7.5	6.1 ± 0.5	1.275	5.5	7.5	6.1 ± 0.5	1.275
RMC 100%	5.5	7.0	6.2 ± 0.4	1.083	5.5	7.0	6.2 ± 0.4	1.083
NOPMEC	5.5	10.4	7.7 ± 1.6	2.204	5.5	9.5	7.6 ± 1.4	1.945
NOPMEC$_{limit}$	5.5	11.5	8.1 ± 1.9	2.525	5.5	10.0	7.8 ± 1.5	2.088

4.2 Results

Table 4.1 lists the NCC values for the performed experiments. For the single sphere datasets, the *Initial* volume shows the best result. All reconstructions using motion compensation and more data have a lower NCC value, although RMC 100% scores higher than RMC 80%. For the sphere grid datasets, RMC 100% has the highest NCC value, followed by both NOPMEC reconstructions. Thus, for the sphere grid datasets, the reconstructions using 100% of the projection data scored best. Comparing the static and in-motion variants of both single sphere and grid datasets, little to no influence of the motion on the NCC value of the motion-compensated reconstructions can be seen.

Table 4.2 lists the shape measurements for the single sphere datasets. In the static case, the FDK reconstruction had the mean diameter value closest to the ground truth (3.6 mm vs. 4 mm), followed by *Initial*. All motion-compensated reconstructions resulted in mean diameters larger than the ground truth. The two NOPMEC reconstructions resulted in very elliptical shapes, with a factor of two between minor and major axis. In the in-motion case, the FDK reconstruction still yielded the best mean diameter. The diameter and eccentricities for all RMC-based reconstructions were identical to those of the static case. The results for the two NOPMEC reconstructions were slightly improved compared to the static case.

Table 4.3: Overall shape measures for sphere grid experiments. Best values are marked in bold.

(a) Static scene.

	Diameter (mm)			e		
	min	max	mean	min	max	mean
FDK	3.2	3.6	**3.4 ± 0.1**	0.177	0.839	**0.432 ± 0.169**
Initial	2.9	3.7	3.3 ± 0.2	0.500	1.053	0.684 ± 0.118
RMC 40 %	3.0	3.7	3.3 ± 0.2	0.530	0.866	0.674 ± 0.106
RMC 80 %	3.1	3.8	**3.4 ± 0.1**	0.177	0.866	0.645 ± 0.191
RMC 100 %	3.2	3.7	**3.4 ± 0.1**	0.177	0.866	0.468 ± 0.161
NOPMEC	2.9	3.9	**3.4 ± 0.2**	0.177	1.031	0.606 ± 0.164
NOPMEC$_{limit}$	2.8	3.9	**3.4 ± 0.2**	0.177	1.031	0.610 ± 0.166

(b) Moving scene.

	Diameter (mm)			e		
	min	max	mean	min	max	mean
FDK	3.2	3.6	**3.5 ± 0.1**	0.177	0.839	0.608 ± 0.177
Initial	2.9	3.7	3.3 ± 0.2	0.468	1.053	0.682 ± 0.118
RMC 40 %	3.0	3.7	3.3 ± 0.2	0.530	0.866	0.670 ± 0.105
RMC 80 %	3.1	3.7	3.4 ± 0.1	0.177	0.866	0.643 ± 0.193
RMC 100 %	3.2	3.7	3.4 ± 0.1	0.177	0.866	**0.494 ± 0.166**
NOPMEC	2.9	3.8	3.4 ± 0.2	0.177	0.935	0.621 ± 0.164
NOPMEC$_{limit}$	2.9	3.8	3.4 ± 0.2	0.177	0.935	0.625 ± 0.159

Table 4.4: Shape measures for centre sphere of sphere grid experiments. Best values are marked in bold.

	Static Scene Diameter (mm)			e	Moving Scene Diameter (mm)			e
	min	max	mean		min	max	mean	
FDK	3.0	3.5	3.4 ± 0.2	**0.468**	2.8	4.2	**3.5 ± 0.3**	0.791
Initial	2.6	3.5	3.2 ± 0.4	0.599	2.6	3.5	3.2 ± 0.4	0.599
RMC 40 %	2.6	3.5	3.2 ± 0.4	0.599	2.6	3.5	3.1 ± 0.4	0.599
RMC 80 %	2.6	3.5	3.2 ± 0.4	0.599	2.6	3.5	3.2 ± 0.4	0.599
RMC 100 %	2.8	3.5	3.3 ± 0.3	0.530	2.8	3.5	3.3 ± 0.3	**0.530**
NOPMEC	2.8	3.5	**3.5 ± 0.2**	0.530	2.8	3.5	3.4 ± 0.3	**0.530**
NOPMEC$_{\text{limit}}$	2.8	3.5	**3.5 ± 0.2**	0.530	2.8	3.5	3.4 ± 0.3	**0.530**

Table 4.3 lists the overall shape measurements for the sphere grid datasets. In the static case, all mean diameters – except for *Initial* and RMC 40 % – were within one voxel size (0.56 mm) of the ground truth, a noticeable difference to the single sphere datasets. The eccentricity value of the FDK reconstruction was lowest, followed by RMC 100 %. A continuous decrease in eccentricity could be observed going from *Initial* to RMC 100 %. In the in-motion case, the diameter measurements were almost identical to the static case. The eccentricity values were also very similar, with the exception of the FDK reconstruction. Therefore RMC 100 % resulted in the lowest eccentricity.

Table 4.4 lists the shape measurements for the central sphere of the sphere grid datasets. In the static case, the NOPMEC reconstructions had the best mean diameter. The central sphere's eccentricity values for all motion-compensated reconstructions were lower than the corresponding overall eccentricities (cf. Table 4.3a). In the in-motion case, only minimal change could be observed in the mean diameter measurements. The same holds for the eccentricity values, except for the FDK reconstruction. Thus, the reconstructions using 100 % of the projection data scored best regarding eccentricity.

Table 4.5 lists the shape measurements for the 98 outer spheres of the sphere grid datasets. In the static case, the RMC 80 % and both NOPMEC reconstructions had the best mean diameter, followed by RMC 100 % and FDK, which were within one voxel size of the ground truth. The FDK reconstruction resulted in the lowest eccentricity value, followed by RMC 100 %. In the in-motion case, the FDK and RMC 80 % reconstructions resulted in the best mean diameters, while the RMC 100 % and both NOPMEC reconstructions were within one voxel size of the ground truth. The RMC 100 % reconstruction had the lowest eccentricity value. In general, the results for the outer spheres were very similar to the overall statistics, keeping in mind that the outer spheres account for 78 % of the total number of spheres in the grid.

Figure 4.4 shows three reconstruction results for the static single sphere dataset. The more elliptical shape and larger size of the RMC 100 % result compared to the RMC 40 % result can clearly be seen, as can be the strongly elliptical shape of the NOPMEC result. Figure 4.5 shows four reconstruction results for the moving single sphere dataset. In the image reconstructed with FDK, the resting position and reversal

Table 4.5: Shape measures for outer spheres of sphere grid experiments. Best values are marked in bold.

(a) Static scene.

	Diameter (mm)			e		
	min	max	mean	min	max	mean
FDK	3.2	3.6	3.4 ± 0.1	0.177	0.839	**0.422 ± 0.179**
Initial	2.9	3.7	3.3 ± 0.2	0.500	1.053	0.684 ± 0.119
RMC 40 %	3.0	3.6	3.3 ± 0.2	0.530	0.866	0.672 ± 0.107
RMC 80 %	3.1	3.8	**3.5 ± 0.1**	0.177	0.866	0.621 ± 0.200
RMC 100 %	3.3	3.7	3.4 ± 0.1	0.177	0.866	0.455 ± 0.176
NOPMEC	3.1	3.9	**3.5 ± 0.2**	0.177	1.031	0.616 ± 0.182
NOPMEC$_{limit}$	3.1	3.9	**3.5 ± 0.2**	0.177	1.031	0.622 ± 0.184

(b) Moving scene.

	Diameter (mm)			e		
	min	max	mean	min	max	mean
FDK	3.2	3.6	**3.5 ± 0.1**	0.177	0.839	0.600 ± 0.178
Initial	2.9	3.7	3.3 ± 0.2	0.500	1.053	0.683 ± 0.118
RMC 40 %	3.0	3.6	3.3 ± 0.2	0.530	0.866	0.668 ± 0.106
RMC 80 %	3.1	3.7	**3.5 ± 0.1**	0.177	0.866	0.619 ± 0.202
RMC 100 %	3.2	3.7	3.4 ± 0.1	0.177	0.866	**0.487 ± 0.183**
NOPMEC	3.0	3.8	3.4 ± 0.2	0.177	0.935	0.632 ± 0.182
NOPMEC$_{limit}$	3.0	3.8	3.4 ± 0.2	0.177	0.935	0.638 ± 0.176

point of the sphere can be identified. This is also reflected by the profile shown in Figure 4.3b, which was taken along the direction of movement. The RMC 40 % result shows a good spherical shape and approximate size, but also the effects of the smooth ramp filter kernel can be seen by the unsharp delineation of the sphere. The RMC 100 % result shows an elliptical shape that is drawn towards the direction of movement, indicating a non-complete motion compensation. The NOPMEC result looks very similar to the static result, i.e. strongly elliptical.

Figure 4.6 shows three reconstruction results for the static sphere grid dataset. The RMC 40 % result shows good size and shape properties, while some artefacts can be seen between the spheres. The RMC 100 % result also shows good size and shape properties, with the artefacts having disappeared. The NOPMEC result displays elliptical deformations of the outer spheres of the grid. Figure 4.7 shows four reconstruction results for the moving sphere grid dataset. Again, in the FDK result, the resting positions and reversal points of the spheres can be identified. The RMC 40 % result looks very similar to the static result, with some artefacts being present between the spheres. Similarly, the observations of the static results for RMC 100 % and NOPMEC also hold for the in-motion results.

4.3 Discussion and Conclusions

In this chapter, a simulation study using a numerical phantom was presented. The phantom either represented a single sphere or a grid of $5 \times 5 \times 5$ spheres floating in free space, each either static or in motion. Simulated projection images were generated using the CONRAD software framework and a trajectory calibrated from a real C-arm imaging system. Seven reconstructions (FDK, *Initial*, RMC 40 %, RMC 80 %, RMC 100 %, NOPMEC, and NOPMEC$_{\text{limit}}$) were generated from every dataset. The *Initial* volume was used as the reference volume for RMC 40 % and NOPMEC/NOPMEC$_{\text{limit}}$. Normalised cross-correlation, diameter measurements and eccentricity were used as metrics to quantify the reconstruction accuracy.

For the single sphere experiments, the non-motion-compensated FDK and *Initial* reconstructions resulted in the best NCC, diameter and eccentricity values in both the static and in-motion case. This leads to three conclusions. For one, the resting phase of the in-motion phantom was long enough to allow for a near-perfect reconstruction of the sphere at that position by simple ECG-gated or even non-gated, non-compensated reconstruction. As Figure 4.5 illustrates, the FDK reconstructions still clearly show a second sphere due to the motion in the dataset. Since the shape metrics were only evaluated at the known resting sphere position, they did not account for this and only evaluated the sphere reconstructed at the resting position. Which is why both the visual impression as well as the quantitative measurements need to be taken into consideration. Finally, all motion-compensated reconstructions suffered from overestimation of the diameter and a non-spherical shape. Since the dataset allows for any kind of motion within the empty areas without penalising either cost function of RMC or NOPMEC, the single sphere datasets seem to present very badly conditioned optimisation problems for both algorithms, with NOPMEC being more affected due to the lower number of spatial B-spline control points. One additional observation was that even the FDK reconstruction of the static dataset resulted in a diameter

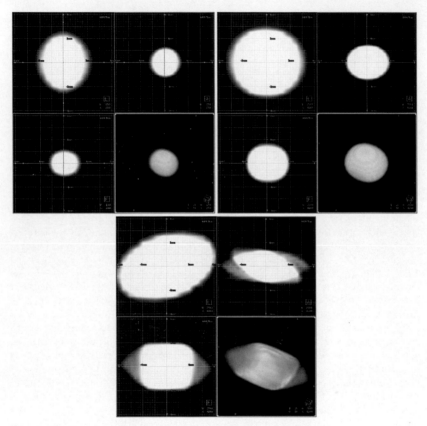

Figure 4.4: Reconstruction results of static single sphere dataset.
Top row: Left RMC 40 %, right RMC 100 %. Bottom row: NOPMEC.

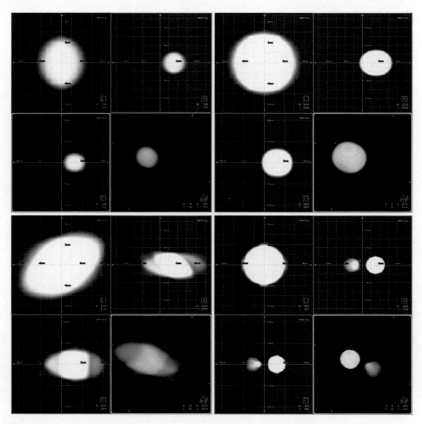

Figure 4.5: Reconstruction results of moving single sphere dataset.
Top row: Left RMC 40 %, right RMC 100 %. Bottom row: Left NOPMEC, right FDK.

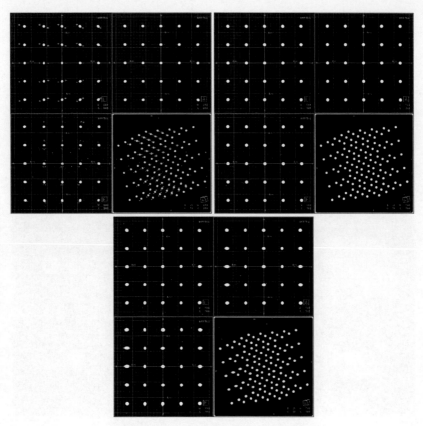

Figure 4.6: Reconstruction results of static sphere grid dataset.
Top row: Left RMC 40 %, right RMC 100 %. Bottom row: NOPMEC.

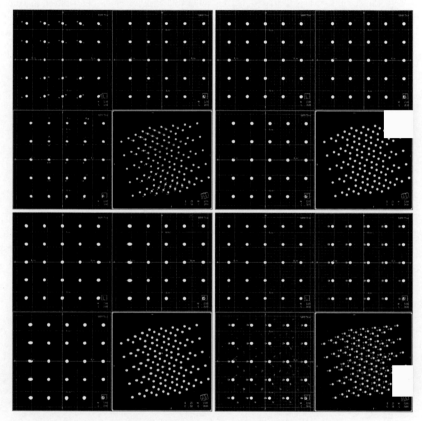

Figure 4.7: Reconstruction results of moving sphere grid dataset.
Top row: Left RMC 40 %, right RMC 100 %. Bottom row: Left NOPMEC, right FDK.

error of 0.4 mm. Since the reconstructed voxel size was 0.56 mm and the spheres had the simulated (high) density of iodine, resulting in partial volume effects, this can be considered to be within measurement accuracy. At the same time, the diameter errors lead to an eccentricity of 0.65 of the baseline reconstruction. This means the eccentricity measure is very sensitive to small diameter variations between the major and minor diameters.

For the sphere grid experiments, RMC 100 % followed by NOPMEC resulted in the best NCC values and RMC 100 % also scored best for the in-motion shape measurements. This contrast to the single sphere case further illustrates the self-regularisation of the motion vector fields when more objects are present in the region of interest and therefore less arbitrary motion vectors are possible. When looking at the central sphere only, all motion-compensated reconstructions except RMC 100 % showed lower eccentricity values for that sphere than over all spheres. Again, the central sphere has the largest number of other spheres around it, regularising the motion vector field. When looking at the outer spheres only, a higher eccentricity compared to the central sphere can be observed for all motion-compensated reconstructions (except RMC 100 %) both quantitatively and qualitatively (cf. Figures 4.6 and 4.7).

No practical difference between the NOPMEC and NOPMEC$_{limit}$ reconstructions could be found. The NOPMEC motion estimation had all possible degrees of freedom of the NOPMEC motion model, while the NOPMEC$_{limit}$ motion estimation only allowed for motion parallel to the current viewing direction at each time point. This means that, for a given time point, motion estimation parallel to the viewing direction is sufficient for motion compensation during backprojection. This strengthens the case for a 2-D–based motion estimation scheme.

A final result of the experiments of this chapter was the establishment of an approximation for the inherent error of the algorithms under investigation. By looking at the results of the static datasets, all present errors can only come from inaccuracies of the image reconstruction process. Thus the results of the static FDK reconstruction represent the baseline quality of the selected cone-beam reconstruction parameters. The additional errors seen in the motion-compensated reconstructions of the static datasets represent the errors introduced by the motion estimation and compensation algorithms.

CAVAREV Simulation Study

In this chapter, the RMC algorithm presented in Chapter 3.1 is evaluated quantitatively using an online evaluation platform called CAVAREV (CArdiac VAsculature Reconstruction EValuation platform). The platform and its metrics are introduced in Section 5.1. The setup of the study is described in Section 5.2. The results are presented in Section 5.3 and discussed in Section 5.4.

Parts of this chapter have been published in [Schw 13b, Schw 13a].

5.1 The CAVAREV Evaluation Platform

CAVAREV [Rohk 10c] is a publicly available online platform for the evaluation of cardiac vasculature reconstruction algorithms. Its aim is to allow fair comparability between algorithms by providing a simulated projection dataset striving for the following properties (from [Rohk 10c]):

- "Anatomical correctness and completeness of the vasculature and its embedding.

- Physiological correctness of the cardiac vasculature motion and its surroundings.

- Acquisition scenario and geometry calibration should correspond to a real-world C-arm system."

A corresponding set of reference 3-D data is used as ground truth for the evaluation step and not made available to the users of the platform.

To achieve these goals, the XCAT phantom [Sega 99, Sega 08] was used to generate two time series of 3-D volumes (the ground truth). One contains only cardiac motion, the other also breathing motion. Both datasets were forward projected using a real-world C-arm acquisition scenario that corresponds to the protocol laid out in Section 1.3. This makes CAVAREV an ideal connection point between the numerical experiments of the last chapter and the clinical study of the next. The projection datasets $\mathcal{D}_C$ (cardiac motion only) and $\mathcal{D}_{BC}$ (additional breathing motion) both consist of 133 projection images showing a thorax and contrasted left and right coronary arteries. Each projection image has a size of 960×960 pixels and an isotropic pixel size of 0.32 mm. More details on the generation of these datasets can be found in [Rohk 10c].

CAVAREV defines two quality measures for 3-D and 4-D reconstruction quality. Since our goal is the reconstruction of a single image volume at a specific reference motion state h_r, we used the 3-D metric introduced as Q_{3D}. For each of the 133 time points (corresponding to the 133 projection images) of the CAVAREV dataset, a static binary volume f_i^{morph} representing the coronary vasculature at the corresponding motion state exists. A reconstruction f submitted to CAVAREV is compared to all 133 ground truth volumes in the following way:

$$Q_i(f) = \max_{a \in \{0,\dots,255\}} \mathrm{dsc}\left(f_i^{\mathrm{morph}}, T(f,a)\right) \quad , \qquad (5.1)$$

where $T(f,a)$ is a threshold function that binarises f at threshold a:

$$T(f,a)(\boldsymbol{x}) = \begin{cases} 1 & , f(\boldsymbol{x}) \geq a \\ 0 & , f(\boldsymbol{x}) < a \end{cases} \quad . \qquad (5.2)$$

The similarity is evaluated using the Dice similarity coefficient

$$\mathrm{dsc}(f_1, f_2) = 2 \frac{\sum_x f_1(x) \cdot f_2(x)}{\sum_x f_1(x) + f_2(x)} \quad , \qquad (5.3)$$

which ranges from 0 (no overlap) to 1 (perfect spatial overlap) since f_1 and f_2 are binary. $Q_i(f)$ is called the motion phase-dependent reconstruction quality. Since CAVAREV accepts reconstructions with 8 bit quantisation, all possible thresholds are tried in this way and the best is used for the quality metric at this time point i. This simulates a manual thresholding operation. The quality measure $Q_{3D} \in [0,1]$ is then computed as

$$Q_{3D}(f) = \max_{i \in \{1,\dots,133\}} Q_i(f) \quad . \qquad (5.4)$$

Again, more details on the quality measures can be found in [Rohk 10c].

5.2   Experimental Setup

Since we assume a strict breath-hold protocol (cf. Sec. 1.3), we used $\mathcal{D}_C$ (cardiac motion only) for the majority of experiments and tested the best-scoring reconstruction parameters on $\mathcal{D}_{BC}$ for reference. We processed the CAVAREV dataset using the parameter set introduced in Section 3.3 and submitted reconstructions with gating window widths $\omega \in \{0.4, 0.8, 1.0\}$, $N_{\mathrm{iter}} \in \{0,1,2,3\}$ and smooth/normal filter kernels to the framework. A study published at the CAVAREV website[1] shows $h_r = 0.9$ to be the optimal reference heart phase for this dataset, so $h_r = 0.9$ was used here

---

[1] http://www.cavarev.com/public-algorithms/algorithm-4, 01.07.2014, no longer online

Table 5.1: CAVAREV results.

ω	N_{iter}	Kernel	Q_{3D}
0.4	*Initial*	smooth	0.742
0.4	*Initial*	normal	0.739
0.4	1	smooth	0.776
0.4	1	normal	0.771
0.4	2	smooth	0.776
0.4	2	normal	0.773
0.8	3	smooth	0.809
0.8	3	normal	0.810
1.0	3	smooth	0.807
1.0	3	normal	0.823

as well. The reconstructed 3-D volumes had an isotropic voxel size of 0.5 mm and a size of 98^3 mm^3.

Since, as mentioned in Section 5.1, the CAVAREV platform only accepts reconstructions with 8 bit quantisation, the reconstructed 16 bit volumes were re-quantised in the following way before being submitted:

$$f^{(8)} = \text{round}\left(255 \cdot \frac{f^{(16)} - \min\left(f^{(16)}\right)}{\max\left(f^{(16)}\right) - \min\left(f^{(16)}\right)}\right) \tag{5.5}$$

5.3 Results

Table 5.1 lists the Q_{3D} values for the different reconstructions generated. For $\omega = 0.4$, all reconstructions with a normal filter kernel scored lower than those with a smooth kernel. The first iteration of RMC improved the Q_{3D} value by 5 %, the second iteration did not change it when using a smooth kernel. A small improvement is seen between 1 iteration / normal and 2 iterations / normal, but the score is still below that of the smooth kernel reconstruction. A third iteration with $\omega = 0.8$ improved the Q_{3D} value by another 4 %, with a slightly better score when using a normal filter kernel. A third iteration with $\omega = 1.0$ improved the Q_{3D} value by another 4 % (smooth) and 6 % (normal). The total improvement of $\omega = 1.0$ / normal over the initial value was 11 %. The published Q_{3D} value for a straight-forward FDK reconstruction is $Q_{\text{3D}} = 0.431^2$. The improvement of $\omega = 1.0$ / normal over FDK was therefore 91 %. For reference, the Q_{3D} value of NOPMEC is $Q_{\text{3D}} = 0.728$ [Rohk 11].

Figure 5.1 shows volume renderings of the best-scoring reconstructions for each algorithm stage. Between $\omega = 0.4$ and $\omega = 0.8$, a clear decrease in artefact level can be observed (as indicated by the arrows). In addition, vessel structures appear more homogeneous with a better visibility of distal parts. The reconstruction with $\omega = 1.0$ shows further improved vessel homogeneity, but also some motion blur.

In Figure 5.2, the effect of smooth vs. normal filter kernel is shown for reconstructions with $\omega = 0.8$ and $\omega = 1.0$. For both, an improved sharpness, resolution and

---

[2] http://www.cavarev.com, 05.01.2018

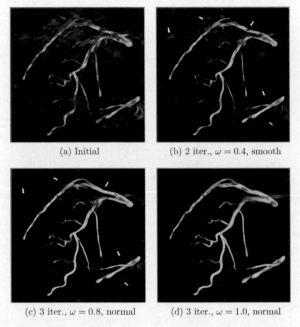

(a) Initial   (b) 2 iter., $\omega = 0.4$, smooth

(c) 3 iter., $\omega = 0.8$, normal   (d) 3 iter., $\omega = 1.0$, normal

Figure 5.1: Reconstruction results of the CAVAREV dataset. The grey scale window width was 1000 HU.

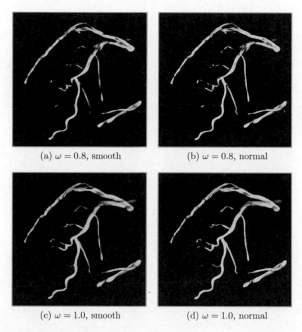

(a) $\omega = 0.8$, smooth   (b) $\omega = 0.8$, normal

(c) $\omega = 1.0$, smooth   (d) $\omega = 1.0$, normal

Figure 5.2: Influence of filter kernel on reconstruction result. The grey scale window width was 1000 HU.

homogeneity is seen. The effect is stronger for $\omega = 1.0$, as expected from the larger Q_{3D} difference between smooth and normal for this gating window width.

Testing the parameter set on dataset $\mathcal{D}_{BC}$ yielded $Q_{3D} = 0.386$, which is considerably lower than for the cardiac motion-only dataset. For reference, settings equivalent to the initial reconstruction (ECG-gated FDK reconstruction with $\omega = 0.4$) result in $Q_{3D} = 0.208^3$ and straight-forward FDK in $Q_{3D} = 0.206^2$. Therefore the improvement over the initial reconstruction was 86 % and over FDK 87 %.

5.4   Discussion and Conclusions

In this chapter, the RMC algorithm was tested using the publicly available evaluation platform CAVAREV. Reconstructions after a different number of iterations and with different filter kernels were submitted to the platform.

Since the cardiac motion of the dataset is strictly periodic, ECG-gating already performs very well. Due to this, the initial reconstruction is already good enough so that all data inconsistencies are removed in the first iteration. A second iteration of RMC does not improve the quality anymore. However, for real clinical data, the initial reconstruction problem can be so badly conditioned that a second iteration is mandatory for a sufficient quality. This will be shown in the following chapters. The Q_{3D} value after one and two iterations was improved by 5 % compared to the initial reconstruction.

From a theoretical viewpoint, $\omega = 0.4$ results in a low number of projections used for reconstruction, promoting undersampling artefacts. These are amplified by a sharper kernel, resulting in a lower score. Therefore, we suggest a more conservative smooth kernel for both the initial and all motion-compensated reconstructions that use a 40 % gating window size.

If a larger gating window is used, an improved reconstruction of the vasculature can be obtained, as shown by the higher Q_{3D} scores. Additionally, a sharper kernel does improve the achievable quality, since undersampling artefacts are not as dominant anymore. In the volume renderings, a clear decrease in undersampling artefacts can be seen in reconstructions with a large gating window. When using all projection data and a normal filter kernel, an improvement of 11 % over the initial reconstruction and 91 % over FDK could be obtained.

The test on dataset $\mathcal{D}_{BC}$ showed a drastic Q_{3D} improvement after motion compensation of 86 % (initial reconstruction) and 87 % (FDK). At the same time, the similar scores of the initial reconstruction and simple FDK demonstrate the ineffectiveness of ECG-gating for highly non-periodic data. Still, the low score of 0.386 when compared to 0.823 for dataset $\mathcal{D}_C$ emphasises the breath-hold requirement of the clinical acquisition protocol.

All RMC results presented here are available online at http://www.cavarev.com/ and were the leading results between their publication in 2013 and the publication of [Taub 17], scoring second and third place at the time of this writing.

The parameter set introduced in Section 3.3 and used throughout this work was established heuristically by previous experience and small-scale studies on few clinical

---

[3]http://www.cavarev.com, 05.01.2018

datasets. The general applicability on (simulated) coronary vasculature data and the validity of filter kernel choices for different ω was demonstrated in this chapter. The algorithm and parameter's fitness for a large set of clinical data will be analysed in the next two chapters.

CHAPTER 6

Human Clinical Study – Quantitative Evaluation

In this chapter, the RMC algorithm presented in Chapter 3.1 and the state-of-the-art algorithm NOPMEC are evaluated quantitatively in a human clinical study. For this purpose, a specialised software tool for the evaluation of coronary vasculature reconstructions was developed in a collaborative effort with Christoph Forman and Jens Wetzl. This software is presented and evaluated in Section 6.1, parts of which have been published in [Schw 14a]. In Section 6.2, the patient population and design of the clinical study are laid out. The results of the study are presented in Section 6.3 and discussed in Section 6.4.

Parts of this chapter have also been published in [Schw 14b].

6.1 CoroEval

A quantification of the effects of motion compensation requires either an observer study or well-defined (possibly automated) metrics. We would like to focus on the second point in this chapter, (semi-)automated evaluation of metrics on reconstructed volumetric datasets. These metrics should reflect properties specific to coronary vasculature. We chose vessel sharpness and diameter, both of which are commonly used in related work (cf. Chapter 2). Sharpness is one of the aspects an observer would consider as the quality of a reconstruction. Vessel diameter is important if 3-D quantitative coronary angiography (QCA) is to be performed afterwards.

An evaluation of 3-D coronary vasculature reconstructions should have the following properties:

1. A standardised method of computing sharpness and diameter of vessels.

2. As little user-dependency as possible. Manual selection of measurement points and vessel profiles limits the number of measurements taken and introduces subjectivity, which should be avoided.

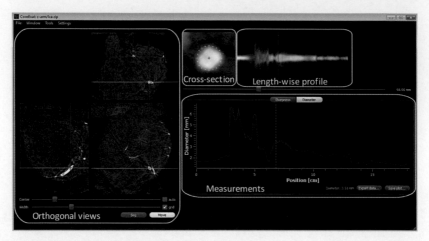

Figure 6.1: Vessel diameter measurements on a C-arm dataset. Yellow annotations were inserted for illustration purposes.

3. Measurements taken on the raw intensity data, without application of display windowing functions.

4. Repeatability by depending on as few parameters in the evaluation algorithm as possible and documenting their values.

From this, we developed the CoroEval software that is described in the remainder of this section. Its purpose is the evaluation of 3-D coronary vessel reconstructions independent of the imaging modality used. So far, we have successfully used it on C-arm CT and MRI data. Early versions of the software were already used for the evaluation in [Picc 12, Schw 13b, Schw 13a, Form 13, Form 14].

6.1.1   Software Overview

CoroEval is built using various open source libraries to ensure multi-platform compatibility and minimise code duplication. Specifically, we make heavy use of the Qt framework[1] for GUI and general application routines and the Qwt widget library[2] for 2-D plotting. Loading of DICOM datasets is supported by the Grassroots DICOM library[3] and libzip[4]. Routines from the Geometric Tools library[5] are used for linear algebra and B-spline curve fitting. Mesh generation and export is supported by the OpenMesh library[6]. Finally, the CMake build system[7] is used for dependency

---

[1]http://qt-project.org/
[2]http://qwt.sourceforge.net/
[3]http://gdcm.sourceforge.net/
[4]http://www.nih.at/libzip/
[5]http://www.geometrictools.com/
[6]http://www.openmesh.org/
[7]http://www.cmake.org/

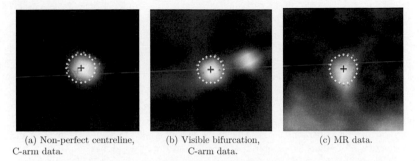

(a) Non-perfect centreline,   (b) Visible bifurcation,   (c) MR data.
C-arm data.   C-arm data.

Figure 6.2: Cross-sectional vessel profile views. Shown are centreline point (blue cross), estimated actual centre (red cross), detected vessel borders (green dots) and estimated vessel diameter (white dots).

tracking and support of various development environments. Binary distributions for Windows, Mac OS X and Linux as well as the source code are offered for download at `http://www5.cs.fau.de/CoroEval/`. All screenshots were taken from the Windows version, but window decorations aside, the software looks and works the same on all platforms.

In the remainder of this section, a typical workflow when using CoroEval is presented and the software's features are discussed. Details on the implemented algorithms are presented in Section 6.1.2.

6.1.1.1   Data Import, Visualisation and Navigation

The first step in analysing a new reconstruction is loading the volumetric dataset into CoroEval. The preferred data format is DICOM. Since DICOM volumes typically consist of one file per slice, loading from either a directory or a ZIP file containing all slices is supported. All necessary properties of the volume can be determined from the DICOM header. Alternatively, raw binary data can be loaded. In this case, volume size, voxel size and data format have to be specified. Finally, direct import of CAVAREV result volumes is supported.

The user is assisted in navigating the dataset by three orthogonal views of the volume (coronary, sagittal and axial, cf. Figure 6.1). Slice-wise scrolling, panning and zooming are supported, as well as changing the grey level display window.

6.1.1.2   Segmentation and Segmentation-dependent Visualisation

Vessel centreline segmentation can either be performed manually in CoroEval, or loaded from disk when another software is used for segmentation. Currently, only a single branch can be examined at one time, since only a non-branching centreline is supported.

For manual segmentation, centreline points can be inserted through the orthogonal volume views. An external centreline segmentation can currently be loaded from plain text files or XML files written by MeVisLab. Volume positions in external segmentations are expected in voxel coordinates. The file format for plain text files is one line per point, with the point's x, y and z positions separated by whitespace. XML files need to contain an XMarkerList, which can e.g. come from MeVisLab's tubular tracking module [Frim 08].

Independent of the segmentation source, the list of centreline points can always be saved in plain text format from CoroEval for later re-use.

When a segmentation is available, further visualisation of the volume data is possible: A cross-sectional profile of the vessel at the current point, and a lengthwise profile along the centreline. The lengthwise profile is also known as curved planar reformation. An enlarged version of three cross-sectional profiles is shown in Figure 6.2. This profile view displays the centreline point and the most probable actual vessel centre (cf. Section 6.1.2.2) together with the detected vessel border and estimated diameter.

The lengthwise profile shows the current position on the centreline with a vertical red marker. In Figure 6.1, a stenosis of the vessel can be clearly seen to the left of the position marker. The current position can be set directly from the profile view to intuitively support the navigation along the vessel. Alternatively, a scrollbar under the profile views can be used to go along the centreline.

6.1.1.3　Measurements

The set of centreline points is fit with a cubic B-spline for a continuous representation (cf. Section 6.1.2.1) and regularly sampled at a configurable interval ($d_{MP} = 1.0\,mm$ by default). At each sampled measurement point, the two main metrics vessel sharpness and diameter are evaluated and the results are displayed as a function of position along the centreline (cf. Figure 6.1). The current position is shown as a blue, dashed vertical bar. Both metrics are based on ideas presented in [Li 01], but automated and made more robust by outlier detection. Details on the implementation are given in Section 6.1.2.1. Like the lengthwise profile, the diameter plot also clearly depicts the stenosis in Figure 6.1.

For the analysis of whole vessel segments, an evaluation dialogue is provided (cf. Figure 6.3). After the start and end point of the evaluation are entered, mean sharpness and diameter over the selected region are displayed together with their standard deviations.

6.1.1.4　Measurement Data Export

All plots in CoroEval (vessel sharpness and diameter, individual profile lines) have export functions that allow saving the plot as a bitmap or vector graphic. This enables the direct integration of measurement results into scientific publications. Figure 6.4b was created using this function (with manual annotations). Additionally, the raw measurement data the plot is based on can be exported in text format for further processing in other software.

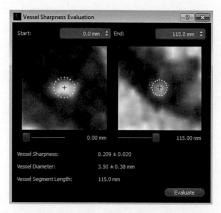

Figure 6.3: Evaluation dialogue, MR data.

6.1.2 Methods

6.1.2.1 Measurement Process

Measurement point interpolation and profile generation. The set of centre-line points is smoothed with a Gaussian kernel ($\sigma = 1.0$, size 3) and fit with a cubic B-spline for an analytical representation of the centreline. This curve is sampled at an interval of $d_{\mathrm{MP}} = 1.0$ mm to get the individual measurement points $\boldsymbol{p}_i \in \mathbb{R}^3, i = 1, 2, \ldots, \frac{\text{seg. length (mm)}}{d_{\mathrm{MP}}}$ at which measurements take place. At each $\boldsymbol{p}_i$, the plane P_i normal to the curve's tangent is computed. Within this plane, $n_{\mathrm{N}} = 10$ equally spaced radial profile lines $L_{i,j}, j = 1, 2, \ldots, n_{\mathrm{N}}$ of length $l_{\mathrm{profile}} = 21$ mm through $\boldsymbol{p}_i$ are created. Figure 6.4a illustrates this for five measurement points. Each profile line $L_{i,j}$ is a 1-D representation of (original 16 bit, non-windowed, 2× linearly oversampled) voxel intensities along its length. There is a dialogue window to inspect the individual $L_{i,j}$ for a given $\boldsymbol{p}_i$, including the detected points of interest, as described in the next two sections.

Extrema detection. Extremal points of the profile line $L_{i,j}$ are detected using finite differences of a smoothed version of $L_{i,j}$ (Gaussian kernel with $\sigma = 1.0$, size 5). A plateau is assumed if $\|\nabla L_{i,j,\mathrm{smooth}}\| < t_{\mathrm{plateau}}$, where $t_{\mathrm{plateau}} = 15$ is a heuristic noise-dependent threshold. The actual extrema positions are searched in (non-smoothed) $L_{i,j}$ within the Gaussian kernel size around the detected positions. From all resulting extrema, and by going along the list of detected maxima, a list of minimum/maximum/minimum tuples is built while ensuring a minimum–minimum distance of at least $d_{\mathrm{min-min}} = 1$ mm. Possible non-unique tuples (i.e. multiple minima candidates for one maxima) are taken care of by building multiple tuples. If no valid pairs are found, the profile line is not considered further. To correct for noise-related local minima, the smaller minimum–maximum magnitude needs to be at least $t_{\mathrm{minmax}} = 0.5$ of the larger magnitude. From all remaining tuples, the one with its

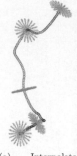

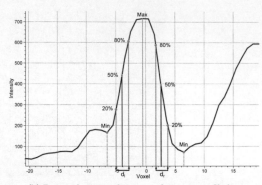

(a)   Interpolated
measurement points
and   example   pro-
file   lines   along   a
centreline.

(b) Detected points of interest along one profile line.

Figure 6.4: Measurement process.

maximum closest to the centre of the profile line is returned as the extrema tuple for
this profile line.

Vessel sharpness.   For each profile line $L_{i,j}$, six points of interest are defined using
the extrema tuple of this line (cf. Figure 6.4b): left minimum, 20% and 80% points,
maximum, and right 80%, 20% and minimum points. Let d_l and d_r be the distances
in mm between the respective 20% and 80% points. Both d_l and d_r depend on i and
j, which is omitted for readability. Vessel sharpness for $L_{i,j}$ is then [Li 01]:

$$s_{i,j} = \frac{2}{d_l + d_r} . \tag{6.1}$$

The advantage of using this 20%–80% edge-rise distance instead of the minimum–maximum distance as a measure of sharpness is the independence from the
vessel diameter.

For the measurement point p_i, vessel sharpness can be defined as the average of
its individual $s_{i,j}$:

$$s_i = \frac{1}{n_N} \sum_{j=1}^{n_N} s_{i,j} \tag{6.2}$$

Since misdetection of extrema can never be fully avoided in real data, two outlier
detections take place in the actual calculation of s_i:

1. If $L_{i,j}$ did not generate valid extrema pairs (cf. Section 6.1.2.1 – **Extrema
   Detection**), its $s_{i,j}$ is not used in Equation 6.2.

2. First, s_i is calculated as in Equation 6.2 (excluding invalid $L_{i,j}$) while also
   calculating the standard deviation σ over all $s_{i,j}$. Then s_i is calculated again,
   while excluding all $s_{i,j} > 2 \cdot \sigma$.

Algorithm 6.1: Diameter estimation.

Input: Profile lines $L_{i,j}$ at p_i
Output: Diameter d_i

1 Build a list valid of all $L_{i,j}$ that generated valid extrema pairs
2 **if** empty(valid) **then**
3 | **return** $d_i \leftarrow 0$
4 **end**
   /* Let $d_{i,j}$ be the distance between the 50 % points of profile $L_{i,j}$
      */
5 $m_d \leftarrow$ median$(d_{i,j}, j \in$ valid$)$, $\sigma_d \leftarrow$ stddev$(d_{i,j}, j \in$ valid$)$
   /* $\mathbf{Max}_{i,j} \in \mathbb{R}^3$ are the volume coordinates of the detected maximum
      of profile $L_{i,j}$.   */
6 $m_{\max} \leftarrow$ median$(\mathbf{Max}_{i,j}, j \in$ valid$)$, $\sigma_{\max} \leftarrow$ stddev$(\mathbf{Max}_{i,j}, j \in$ valid$)$
7 **foreach** $j \in$ valid **do**
8 | **if** $|d_{i,j} - m_d| > 2 \cdot \sigma_d$ **then**
9 | | remove j from valid and **continue**
10 | **end**
11 | **if** $\|Max_{i,j} - m_{max}\| > 2 \cdot \sigma_{max}$ **then**
12 | | remove j from valid and **continue**
13 | **end**
14 **end**
15 **if** empty(valid) **then**
16 | **return** $d_i \leftarrow 0$
17 **end**
18 Fit an ellipse to the 2-D coordinates (in plane P_i) of the 50 % points in valid
    [Hali 98]
19 **if** *fitting fails* **then**
20 | **return** $d_i \leftarrow 0$
21 **end**
   /* Let a,b be the radii in mm of the ellipse. Return the diameter
      of a circle of the same area as the ellipse.   */
22 **return** $d_i \leftarrow 2\sqrt{a \cdot b}$

Vessel diameter. As shown in Figure 6.4b, two additional points of interest are defined along each profile $L_{i,j}$: left and right 50 % points between minimum and maximum. Their distances $d_{i,j}$ are used for the diameter estimation, assuming that the diameter along one profile corresponds to the full width at half between minima and maximum. Since vessels can be elliptical (especially in motion-compensated reconstruction with bad motion estimation), this should be taken into account. In addition, outlier detection is performed. This leads to the procedure for diameter estimation at a measurement point p_i outlined in Algorithm 6.1. Over all valid profile lines $L_{i,j}$, the median and standard deviation of $d_{i,j}$ are calculated. In addition, the median 3-D coordinate of the detected maxima and their standard deviation are calculated. These values are used for outlier detection. If either a $d_{i,j}$ differs more than two standard deviations from the median, or a maximum coordinate is further away than two standard deviations from the median coordinate, then the corresponding profile line $L_{i,j}$ is removed from the list of valid profiles. If there are no remaining valid profiles, the algorithm returns 0. Otherwise, the 2-D (in plane P_i) coordinates of the remaining 50 % points are passed to a numerically stable ellipse fitting algorithm. We used the algorithm from [Hali 98] in CoroEval, which is an improved version of the algorithm presented in [Fitz 96]. Finally, the returned diameter is that of a circle with the same area as the estimated ellipse:

$$d_i = 2\sqrt{a \cdot b} \, , \tag{6.3}$$

where a and b are the major and minor radius (in mm) of the ellipse.

This approach of assuming an elliptical vessel cross-section and expressing its diameter as the diameter of a circle with equivalent area was chosen to be similar to clinically established methods for 3-D quantitative coronary angiography [Onum 11, Suzu 13]. If the algorithm fails and returns 0, the average diameter

$$d_i = \frac{1}{n_N} \sum_{j=1}^{n_N} d_{i,j} \tag{6.4}$$

is used. The average diameter is only calculated over valid profile lines.

Post-processing. Vessel sharpness and diameter values along the whole set of measurement points are median filtered with a kernel size of 3 to reduce noise-related influences.

6.1.2.2 Segmentation Correction

Since neither a manual nor a (semi-)automatic segmentation guarantee a perfect centreline extraction, the need for a segmentation correction can arise. We make use of the cross-sectional planes P_i to offer both manual interaction and an automated correction.

Manual interaction. When enabled from the tools menu, the user can click into the currently displayed cross-sectional plane and redefine the in-plane location of the measurement point p_i. This is especially useful if the current location is completely

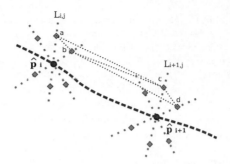

Figure 6.5: Illustration of the mesh creation method. The blue dashed line represents the centreline. Two vessel centre points $\hat{\boldsymbol{p}}_i$ and $\hat{\boldsymbol{p}}_{i+1}$ are shown as red dots along the centreline. At each vessel centre point, three profile lines L are drawn. Along each profile line, the left and right 50 % points are indicated as green square markers. The resulting two triangles from two subsequent point pairs are outlined with black dots.

outside of the vessel, where an automated correction may not converge to the right position. In consequence, after manual correction, the distance between measurement points may be different from the initial 1 mm.

Automated correction.   Even if $\boldsymbol{p}_i$ is not in the centre of the vessel, the vessel boundaries are reliably detected as the 50 % points of interest (cf. Section 6.1.2.1 – **Vessel Diameter**) in many cases, as long as the profile line is long enough to actually contain the boundaries. For every profile line $L_{i,j}$ we can therefore compute the assumed vessel centre $\hat{\boldsymbol{p}}_{i,j} \in \mathbb{R}^3$ as the midpoint between both 50% points. Since the location of $L_{i,j}$ in plane P_i and the location of P_i in the volume are known, the calculation of the 3-D position of the assumed vessel centre from its 1-D position along $L_{i,j}$ is trivial. The most probable actual vessel centre location $\hat{\boldsymbol{p}}_i \in \mathbb{R}^3$ is then the centre of mass of all $\hat{\boldsymbol{p}}_{i,j}$. This process can be repeated until no changes larger than the volume's voxel size take place. In our experiments, we found a typical convergence in less than 10 iterations. The user can select this correction either only for the current measurement point or for all points. Figure 6.2a shows an example of $\boldsymbol{p}_i$ vs. $\hat{\boldsymbol{p}}_i$ before automated correction of $\boldsymbol{p}_i$.

6.1.2.3   Mesh Generation and Export

Vessel segmentations can be exported as a centreline point cloud, vessel surface point cloud (consisting of the 50 % points) or vessel surface mesh. The first two options simply save the raw point lists for further processing with other applications. The third option allows visualising the vessel lumen segmentation mesh or using it for further analysis, e.g. fluid simulations. How the surface mesh is generated is explained in the remainder of this section. The OpenMesh software library used in CoroEval includes a 3-D mesh viewer that complements the mesh export in CoroEval with visualisation features.

Since the vessel lumen segmentation introduced in Section 6.1.2.1 already implicitly returns the vessel topology along the centreline, mesh generation is reduced to the problem of finding surface point correspondences. The procedure described in the remainder of this section is illustrated in Figure 6.5. To generate a surface mesh, we first create a list of points on the surface of the vessel for each $\hat{p}_i$. Let $v_{i,j}^{(\ell)}$ and $v_{i,j}^{(r)}$ denote the left and right 50 % points of profile line $L_{i,j}$. The list $V_i = \left[v_{i,1}^{(\ell)}, \ldots, v_{i,n_\mathrm{N}}^{(\ell)}, v_{i,1}^{(r)}, \ldots, v_{i,n_\mathrm{N}}^{(r)}\right]$ then already contains the topological information for the vessel surface points on the ring around the centreline point $\hat{p}_i$.

Outlier points are detected in two steps (cf. Algorithm 6.1 and Section 6.1.2.2): 1. If the distance of $\hat{p}_{i,j}$ to $\hat{p}_i$ differs by more than two standard deviations from the average distance over all profile lines, then $v_{i,j}^{(\ell)}$ and $v_{i,j}^{(r)}$ are marked as outliers. 2. If the distance of $v_{i,j}^{(\ell)}$ or $v_{i,j}^{(r)}$ to $\hat{p}_{i,j}$ differs by more than two standard deviations from the median radius for all surface points in V_i, then $v_{i,j}^{(\ell)}$ or $v_{i,j}^{(r)}$ is also marked as an outlier.

If an outlier $v_{i,j}^{(\ell)}$ or $v_{i,j}^{(r)}$ is surrounded by two inliers on either side, it is replaced by the intersection of the profile line $L_{i,j}$ with a least-squares parabola fit of the inliers. Otherwise, it is replaced by the intersection of the profile line $L_{i,j}$ with a circle of diameter d_i around $\hat{p}_i$.

In the last step, topological information between subsequent surface point lists V_i and V_{i+1} is established by finding an offset o_i such that the summed distance of points $\sum_j \|V_{i,j} - V_{i+1,j+o_i}\|$ is minimised, where indices $j > n_\mathrm{N}$ wrap around. The orientation of the profile lines $L_{i,j}$ around $\hat{p}_i$ is not pre-defined in our method. Therefore, this minimisation finds the rotation of two subsequent surface cross-sections that creates the best-fitting mesh point correspondences.

For two subsequent point pairs $[a, c] = [V_{i,j}, V_{i+1,j+o_i}]$ and $[b, d] = [V_{i,j+1}, V_{i+1,j+o_i+1}]$, two triangles $\triangle acd$ and $\triangle adb$ are added to the mesh (cf. Figure 6.5).

If the actual intensity-based lumen segmentation is not required, but the equivalent diameter d_i around $\hat{p}_i$ fulfils the needs for further processing, there is another option of exporting a vessel surface mesh consisting of circles with diameter d_i around $\hat{p}_i$. This creates a much smoother looking mesh that allows to clearly visualise the properties of the examined vessel. This mesh might also be sufficient for simulations, depending on the complexity of the used physical model.

Figure 6.6 shows an example mesh exported with the described algorithm and visualised with the OpenMesh viewer. For reference, the corresponding diameter curve is also shown. Both the proximal stenosis of this LCX main branch and the distal bifurcation can be clearly seen in both meshes. As mentioned above, the equivalent diameter-based mesh looks smoother than the actual lumen mesh, but both distinct features and general appearance of the vessel are still clearly depicted.

6.1.3   Evaluation

We acquired three phantom datasets on a Siemens zee bi-plane angiographic C-arm device (Siemens Healthcare GmbH, Forchheim, Germany) to evaluate the diameter measurement process (cf. Table 6.1). All acquired projection images had a size of $1240{\times}960$ pixels with an isotropic pixel size of $0.308\,\mathrm{mm}$ ($40{\times}30\,\mathrm{cm}$ detector). Source-

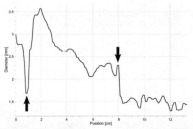

(a) Diameter curve as exported from CoroEval.

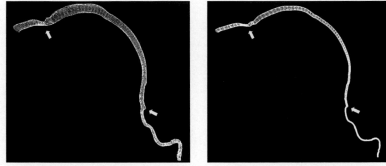

(b) Actual lumen segmentation mesh.   (c) Equivalent diameters mesh.

Figure 6.6: Exported surface meshes for a LCX main branch (visualised with the OpenMesh viewer) and corresponding diameter curve for reference. Arrows indicate stenosis and bifurcation.

Table 6.1: Acquisition parameters for the evaluation datasets.

Dataset	#Proj.	Focal spot (mm)	kVp	Dose/image (µGy)	Voxel size (mm)
M	133	0.7	60	0.36	0.46
T1	133	0.7	90	0.36	0.42
T2	496	0.4	70	1.2	0.39

Table 6.2: Objects used for evaluation.

Object	Dataset	Material	Diameter (mm)	QCA result (mm)
Bar 1	M	Steel	6	6.23±0.03
Bar 2	M	Steel	3	3.06±0.04
Tube	T1, T2	Silicone/contrast	1.5 (inner)	1.55±0.07

Table 6.3: CoroEval results.

Object	Dataset	Diameter (mm)
Bar 1	M	6.25±0.06
Bar 2	M	3.06±0.04
Tube	T1	1.48±0.03
Tube	T2	1.51±0.06

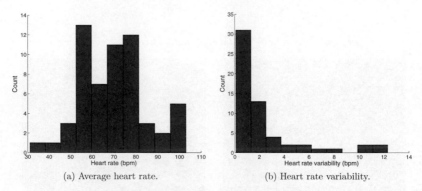

(a) Average heart rate.   (b) Heart rate variability.

Figure 6.7: Heart rate distribution over the patient population.

detector-distance was ∼120 cm with a source-isocentre-distance of ∼80 cm. Dataset M contained two steel bars (bar 1 and bar 2). Datasets T1 and T2 contained a silicone tube filled with contrast agent (iodine concentration 400 mg/ml) and submerged in a water basin. Reference diameters, as given by the manufacturers, and as measured from X-ray fluoroscopy with quantitative coronary angiography (QCA) software, are given in Table 6.2. The QCA software used was from the *syngo* Workplace – Angio/Quant package (Siemens Healthcare GmbH, Forchheim, Germany). From the acquisition geometry, a theoretical resolution at iso-centre of $\frac{80}{120} \cdot 0.308\,\text{mm} \approx 0.21\,\text{mm}$ can be calculated.

All datasets were reconstructed to 3-D volumes (cf. Table 6.1 for isotropic voxel sizes), the object centrelines were segmented semi-automatically [Frim 08] using MeVis-Lab (MeVis Medical Solutions AG, Bremen, Germany), and diameter measurements were taken in CoroEval. Table 6.3 lists the results. The average deviation between QCA and CoroEval was 0.03±0.03 mm. Due to blooming and beam hardening effects, diameter deviations are higher for bar 1 than for bar 2, which was expected.

6.2   Study Outline

6.2.1   Patient Population

For this study, 58 patient datasets from two clinical sites (St. Marienhospital Hamm, Germany and University of Utah Hospital, Salt Lake City, USA) were used. All pa-

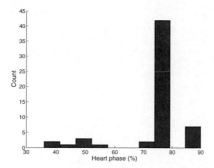

Figure 6.8: Reconstructed heart phase distribution over all datasets.

tients underwent regular diagnostic coronary angiography. Additionally, an acquisition according to the protocol outlined in Section 1.3 was performed for retrospective 3-D reconstruction of either the left or the right coronary artery.

In total, 39 left and 19 right coronary artery datasets fulfilling the clinical protocol were used for this study. No further selection was performed. The statistical distribution of patient heart rates during the acquisition is shown in Figure 6.7. The median heart rate was 71 bpm, the median heart rate variability was 1.3 bpm. With variability, we denote the standard deviation of the heart rate during the acquisition. For an analysis of the influence of heart rate (HR) on motion estimation, patients were further grouped into:

1. Low heart rate: HR < 60 bpm (18 patients)

2. Medium heart rate: 60 bpm $\leq$ HR < 75 bpm (18 patients)

3. High heart rate HR $\geq$ 75 bpm (22 patients).

For an analysis of the influence of heart rate variability (HRV) on motion estimation, patients were further grouped into

1. Low heart rate variability: HRV < 5 bpm (50 patients)

2. High heart rate variability: HRV $\geq$ 5 bpm (8 patients).

6.2.2   Evaluation Protocol

Both algorithms used in this study require the selection of a reference heart phase h_r at which reconstruction shall be carried out. Two reconstructions were generated with the NOPMEC algorithm: One with a fixed $h_r = 0.75$ (end diastole) and one using the automatic heart phase selection algorithm presented in [Rohk 11]. By visual inspection, the heart phase of the reconstruction with better image quality was used for this dataset. Figure 6.8 shows the distribution of the chosen h_r over all datasets. The median h_r was 0.75, which is consistent with findings in previous work [Desj 04, Schw 13b, Schw 13a].

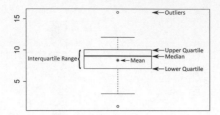

Figure 6.9: Boxplot legend.

After selecting h_r, five reconstructions were generated and evaluated for every dataset:

1. *Initial*: ECG-gated reconstruction without motion compensation ($\omega = 0.4$, $a = 4$, $N_{\text{ign}} = 3$, smooth ramp filter kernel). This also serves as the reference volume for the NOPMEC algorithm.

2. RMC 40 %: Motion-compensated reconstruction with 2 iterations ($\omega = 0.4$, $a = 4$, $N_{\text{ign}} = 3$, smooth ramp filter kernel).

3. RMC 80 %: Motion-compensated reconstruction with 3 iterations ($\omega = 0.8$, $a = 4$, $N_{\text{ign}} = 3$, normal ramp filter kernel).

4. RMC 100 %: Motion-compensated reconstruction with 3 iterations ($\omega = 1.0$, $a = 0$, $N_{\text{ign}} = 0$, normal ramp filter kernel).

5. NOPMEC: Motion-compensated reconstruction ($\omega = 1.0$, $a = 0$, $N_{\text{ign}} = 0$, normal ramp filter kernel).

All volumes were reconstructed to an isotropic voxel size of 0.5 mm. The selected gating window size resulted in the use of 45–56 projection images for the initial reconstruction.

Each reconstruction was then evaluated quantitatively for vessel segmentation length, sharpness and diameter using CoroEval. Vessel segmentation length is implicitly given by the length of the centreline that could be extracted reliably. Additionally, a qualitative evaluation in an observer study was performed, which is presented in the next chapter. MeVisLab's tubular tracking module [Frim 08] was used to generate semi-automatic vessel segmentations for all reconstructions. Runtime and convergence statistics of the algorithms were collected on a workstation with two Intel® Xeon® E5540 CPUs (2.53 GHz) with 16 threads in total and 16 GB of memory. The graphics hardware was an NVIDIA® Quadro® FX 5800 GPU with 4 GB of graphics memory.

6.2.3   Statistical Analysis

The statistical distribution of the evaluation results is mostly shown in boxplots in this work (cf. Figure 6.9). The box contains the middle 50% of all values (interquartile range IQR). Within the box, the median is shown by a thick line, the mean by a star.

The whiskers extend to the last data value within $1.5 \cdot$ IQR of the box. More extreme values (probable outliers) are shown as circles. Average values in tables and text are given as mean ± standard deviation.

Statistical significance of the difference of the means of two distributions was tested with t-tests. Since all five reconstructions for a specific dataset were generated from the same projection data, paired t-tests with Bonferroni correction [Shaf 95] for multiple testing were used. To satisfy the normal distribution assumption of t-tests, quantile–quantile plots (Q–Q plots) are shown for visual inspection of "reasonable similarity" to normally distributed data [Cham 83]. In a Q–Q plot, the statistical quantiles of the measurements are plotted against those of a normal distribution with the same mean and standard deviation. For normally distributed data, all samples lie on the line indicating the quantiles of the normal distribution. We indicate statistical significance with $\star\star\star$ for $p \leq 0.001$, $\star\star$ for $p \leq 0.01$ and $\star$ for $p \leq 0.05$. A $\circ$ indicates $p > 0.05$, i.e. the null hypothesis "no significant difference of the means" cannot be rejected with an error probability of less than 5 %.

6.3   Results

6.3.1   Vessel Segmentation

Successful segmentation of all five reconstructions per dataset was possible for 32 LAD, 31 LCX and 15 RCA, which amounts to ~80 % of all data. Only these datasets were used for further quantitative evaluation to ensure the same amount of observations for all five reconstructions.

For the remaining 20 %, segmentation was possible as follows:

- For 1 LAD, 3 LCX and 2 RCA: Only the *Initial* reconstruction could not be segmented.

- For 1 RCA: *Initial* and NOPMEC could not be segmented.

- For 1 LAD: *Initial*, RMC 40 % and NOPMEC could not be segmented.

- For 5 LAD, 5 LCX and 1 RCA: No segmentation possible at all.

Further investigation of the datasets where no segmentation was possible showed: One patient had a total occlusion of the LAD, which blocks contrast agent from reaching the vessel, making reconstruction impossible. All other LCA datasets where no segmentation was possible had incomplete contrasting of the vessels either at the end of or during the whole acquisition. No apparent contrast problems were found for the one RCA dataset without any segmentation success. The reason for segmentation failure remains unknown for this dataset.

The length of the segmented vessel centreline can be a first indication of reconstruction quality [Li 01]. Even with bad motion compensation, large proximal vessel can often be reconstructed and segmented successfully. But small distal vessel are more difficult. Therefore, we measured the length of the centreline of each segmented reconstruction. Since the achievable length depends on the patient, a relative, normalised length within each dataset was established by subtracting the mean length of

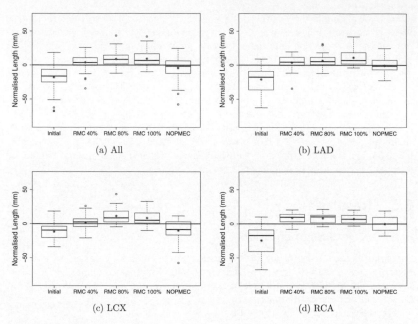

Figure 6.10: Relative length of segmented vessel centrelines. The red line denotes the zero line, which is the average segmentation length over all five reconstructions.

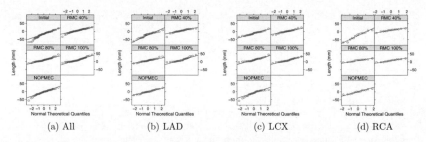

Figure 6.11: Q–Q plots of the distributions of relative segmentation lengths.

Table 6.4: Significance of differences in segmentation lengths.

(a) All

	Initial	40 %	80 %	100 %
40 %	★ ★ ★			
80 %	★ ★ ★	○		
100 %	★ ★ ★	★	○	
NOPMEC	★ ★ ★	★★	★ ★ ★	★ ★ ★

(b) LAD

	Initial	40 %	80 %	100 %
40 %	★ ★ ★			
80 %	★ ★ ★	○		
100 %	★ ★ ★	○	○	
NOPMEC	★ ★ ★	○	○	★

(c) LCX

	Initial	40 %	80 %	100 %
40 %	★★			
80 %	★ ★ ★	★		
100 %	★ ★ ★	○	○	
NOPMEC	○	○	★ ★ ★	★★

(d) RCA

	Initial	40 %	80 %	100 %
40 %	★ ★ ★			
80 %	★ ★ ★	○		
100 %	★	○	○	
NOPMEC	○	○	○	○

all five reconstructions from the individual measurements. The results are shown in Figure 6.10. Over all datasets, NOPMEC represented the average segmentation length, with the exception of LCX segmentations, where it was on the level of the *Initial* reconstruction (Figure 6.10c). *Initial* always represented the shortest segmentation length. The remaining three reconstructions resulted in above-average segmentation lengths, with a slight advantage of RMC 80 % and RMC 100 % over RMC 40 % except for the RCA segmentations (Figure 6.10d).

Figure 6.11 shows the Q–Q plots for the segmentation length measurements. *Initial* and NOPMEC deviate from a normal distribution in the lower tail, while the other distributions display reasonable similarity to a normal distribution. Table 6.4 lists the results of the t-tests, which correspond well to the observations from the boxplots.

6.3.2 Vessel Sharpness

Figure 6.12 shows the results of the vessel sharpness measurements. The same order can be observed for all datasets and sub-groups: RMC 80 % resulted in the sharpest reconstruction, followed by RMC 100 %. RMC 40 % and NOPMEC were very similar in sharpness, although NOPMEC was reconstructed with a normal and RMC 40 % with a smooth kernel. *Initial* always yielded the least sharp reconstruction. Regarding the influence of vessel type, the results indicate slightly less sharp vessels for the LCX than for the LAD. The sharpness of the RCA reconstructions was distinctively lower than the sharpness of LCA reconstructions.

Figure 6.13 shows the Q–Q plots for the vessel sharpness measurements. All distributions display a reasonable similarity to a normal distribution. Table 6.5 lists the results of the t-tests. The observation that RMC 40 % and NOPMEC exhibited very similar sharpness is confirmed. Only over all datasets could a significant difference be found. For the difference between RMC 40 % and RMC 100 %, a significant difference could only be found over all datasets and for the LAD sub-group.

Figure 6.14 shows the vessel sharpness results over all vessel segments grouped by heart rate. The relative ordering between reconstructions is similar to the non-

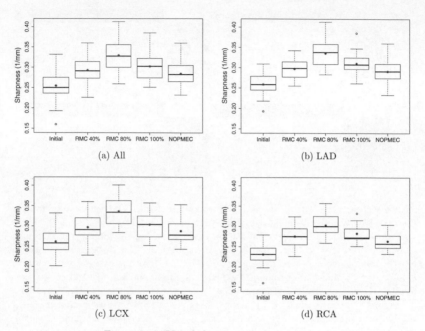

(a) All   (b) LAD

(c) LCX   (d) RCA

Figure 6.12: Vessel sharpness measurements.

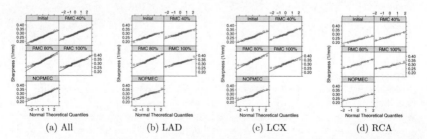

(a) All   (b) LAD   (c) LCX   (d) RCA

Figure 6.13: Q–Q plots of the distributions of vessel sharpness measurements.

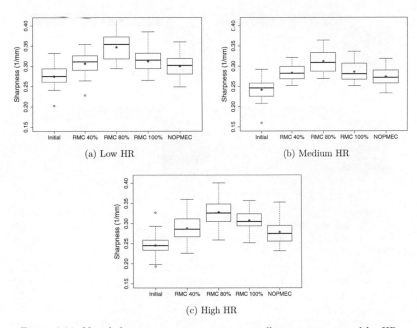

Figure 6.14: Vessel sharpness measurements over all segments grouped by HR.

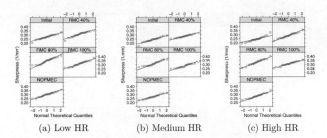

Figure 6.15: Q–Q plots of the distributions of vessel sharpness measurements grouped by HR.

Table 6.5: Significance of differences in vessel sharpness measurements.

(a) All

	Initial	40 %	80 %	100 %
40 %	★★★			
80 %	★★★	★★★		
100 %	★★★	★★★	★★★	
NOPMEC	★★★	★★	★★★	★★★

(b) LAD

	Initial	40 %	80 %	100 %
40 %	★★★			
80 %	★★★	★★★		
100 %	★★★	★★★	★★★	
NOPMEC	★★★	○	★★★	★★★

(c) LCX

	Initial	40 %	80 %	100 %
40 %	★★★			
80 %	★★★	★★★		
100 %	★★★	○	★★★	
NOPMEC	★★★	○	★★★	★★

(d) RCA

	Initial	40 %	80 %	100 %
40 %	★★★			
80 %	★★★	★★★		
100 %	★★★	○	★★★	
NOPMEC	★★★	○	★★★	★★

grouped results. The highest sharpness was achieved in the low HR group (Figure 6.14a). Sharpness in the medium HR group (Figure 6.14b) is distinctively lower, while it is increased again in the high HR group (Figure 6.14c) for RMC 80 % and RMC 100 %.

Figure 6.15 shows the Q–Q plots for the vessel sharpness results grouped by heart rate. All distributions display a reasonable similarity to a normal distribution. Table 6.6 lists the results of the t-tests. In the low HR group, no significant difference between RMC 40 %, RMC 100 % and NOPMEC could be found. In the medium HR group, no significant difference between RMC 40 % and RMC 100 % was found. In the high HR group, no significant difference between RMC 40 % and NOPMEC was found.

Table 6.6: Significance of differences in vessel sharpness measurements grouped by HR.

(a) Low HR

	Initial	40 %	80 %	100 %
40 %	★★★			
80 %	★★★	★★★		
100 %	★★★	○	★★★	
NOPMEC	★★★	○	★★★	○

(b) Medium HR

	Initial	40 %	80 %	100 %
40 %	★★★			
80 %	★★★	★★★		
100 %	★★★	○	★★★	
NOPMEC	★★★	★	★★★	★★★

(c) High HR

	Initial	40 %	80 %	100 %
40 %	★★★			
80 %	★★★	★★★		
100 %	★★★	★★★	★★★	
NOPMEC	★★★	○	★★★	★★★

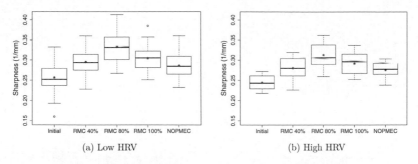

(a) Low HRV   (b) High HRV

Figure 6.16: Vessel sharpness measurements grouped by HRV.

Figure 6.16 shows the vessel sharpness results grouped by heart rate variability. Again, the relative ordering between reconstructions is the same. The maximum sharpness is decreased in the high HRV group, as indicated by the lower top whisker. Overall, the influence of HRV seems to be smaller than that of HR for the investigated datasets. Since the high HRV sub-group consists of only five datasets, no significance tests were performed.

6.3.3   Vessel Diameter

For a comparison of vessel diameters, reference measurements need to be available. We used 2-D QCA (from the *syngo* Workplace – Angio/Quant package (Siemens Healthcare GmbH, Forchheim, Germany)) to estimate reference diameters from suitable 2-D coronary angiography acquisitions. Since an acquisition displaying the desired vessel in good quality and contrast and the corresponding 3-D segmentation for CoroEval need to be available, comparisons could only be made for a subset of all datasets. They were possible for 24 LAD, 25 LCX and 15 RCA (~66 % of all data). We performed repeated 2-D measurements from different angulations for the same vessel if possible. The standard deviation of repeated measurements was 0.14 mm, with a maximum difference of 0.65 mm for one dataset.

Figure 6.17 shows the deviation of measured 3-D diameters from measured 2-D diameters. Over all datasets (Figure 6.17a), the majority of reconstructions displayed less than 0.5 mm deviation. *Initial* resulted in systematically too large vessels, whereas all RMC variants seem to underestimate vessel sizes. NOPMEC on the other hand seems to systematically overestimate vessel sizes. In total, RMC 100 % and NOP-MEC resulted in vessel sizes closest to the measured 2-D diameters, both on average within the standard deviation of the reference measurements. The average diameter deviation of the RMC 40 % reconstructions was worse than RMC 100 % and NOPMEC, but also still barely within the standard deviation of the reference.

Figure 6.18 shows the Q–Q plots for the vessel diameter deviation measurements. For the LCX sub-group, RMC 80 %, RMC 100 % and NOPMEC deviate from a normal distribution in the upper tail. All other distributions display reasonable similarity to a normal distribution. Table 6.7 lists the results of the *t*-tests.

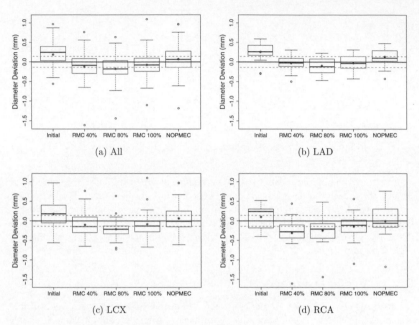

Figure 6.17: Diameter deviation from 2-D QCA measurements. The red line denotes the zero line, i.e. the 2-D QCA reference. The dashed green lines denote the standard deviation of repeated measurements of 2-D QCA.

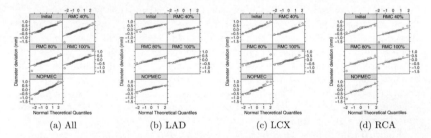

Figure 6.18: Q–Q plots of the distributions of vessel diameter measurements.

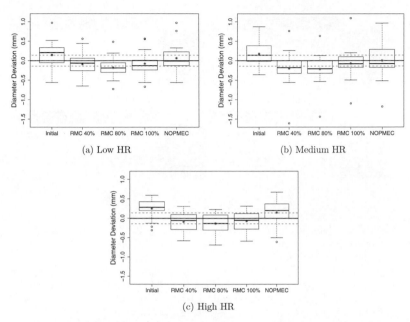

(a) Low HR   (b) Medium HR

(c) High HR

Figure 6.19: Diameter deviation from 2-D QCA measurements grouped by HR. The red line denotes the zero line, i.e. the 2-D QCA reference. The dashed green lines denote the standard deviation of repeated measurements of 2-D QCA.

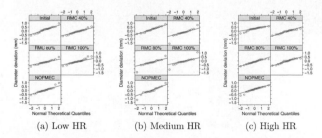

(a) Low HR   (b) Medium HR   (c) High HR

Figure 6.20: Q–Q plots of the distributions of vessel diameter measurements grouped by HR.

Table 6.7: Significance of differences in vessel diameter measurements.

(a) All

	Initial	40 %	80 %	100 %
40 %	★★★			
80 %	★★★	○		
100 %	★★★	○	★★★	
NOPMEC	★★★	★★★	★★★	★★★

(b) LAD

	Initial	40 %	80 %	100 %
40 %	★★★			
80 %	★★★	○		
100 %	★★★	○	○	
NOPMEC	★★	★★★	★★★	★★★

(c) LCX

	Initial	40 %	80 %	100 %
40 %	★★★			
80 %	★★★	★		
100 %	★★	○	★★★	
NOPMEC	★★	★★	★★★	○

(d) RCA

	Initial	40 %	80 %	100 %
40 %	★★			
80 %	★★	○		
100 %	★	★★	★	
NOPMEC	○	★★★	★★★	○

Figure 6.19 shows the diameter deviations grouped by heart rate. It is clearly visible how the diameter error of *Initial* increases with the heart rate. The effect on the compensated reconstructions with RMC is minimal though. NOPMEC is affected most in the high heart rate group.

Figure 6.20 shows the Q–Q plots for the vessel diameter deviations grouped by heart rate. For low HR, the distribution of RMC 100 % has an upper tail. For high HR, the distribution of *Initial* has a lower tail. All other distributions display reasonable similarity to a normal distribution. Table 6.8 lists the results of the *t*-tests.

Table 6.8: Significance of differences in vessel diameter measurements grouped by HR.

(a) Low HR

	Initial	40 %	80 %	100 %
40 %	★★★			
80 %	★★★	○		
100 %	★	○	★★★	
NOPMEC	○	★★★	★★★	○

(b) Medium HR

	Initial	40 %	80 %	100 %
40 %	★★★			
80 %	★★★	○		
100 %	★★★	★★	★★★	
NOPMEC	★	★★★	★★★	○

(c) High HR

	Initial	40 %	80 %	100 %
40 %	★★★			
80 %	★★★	○		
100 %	★★★	○	○	
NOPMEC	○	★★★	★★★	★★

Figure 6.21 shows the diameter deviations grouped by heart rate variability. Again, the diameter error for *Initial* is increased in the high variability group, while the RMC reconstructions are not affected much. For NOPMEC, the median deviation

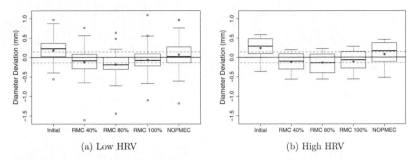

(a) Low HRV   (b) High HRV

Figure 6.21: Diameter deviation from 2-D QCA measurements grouped by HRV. The red line denotes the zero line, i.e. the 2-D QCA reference. The dashed green lines denote the standard deviation of repeated measurements of 2-D QCA.

changes from around zero in the low variability group to slightly outside of the standard deviation of the reference in the high variability group.

6.3.4   Algorithm Convergence and Runtime

In this section, only the runtime behaviour of RMC 100 % is analysed. RMC 40 % corresponds to stopping after two iterations, whereas RMC 80 % corresponds to a third iteration with 80 % of the projection images. Since the registration step is responsible for most of the algorithm runtime [Schw 13b], it is studied in detail here. An overview of the runtime of the other components is given at the end of this section. A short overview of the runtime for NOPMEC is also given at the end of this section for comparison.

Figure 6.22 shows the number of optimisation steps on each resolution level for iterations 1 and 2, i.e. with a gating window size of $\omega = 0.4$. The initial alignment on the lowest resolution level behaved very similarly both between LCA and RCA and between iteration 1 and 2. On the second resolution level, an increase in the number of steps needed can be seen for iteration 2. While the median step count is very similar between iteration 1 and 2, the top range of values is strongly increased. This effect is not as strong for the third resolution level (with M_{spline}), but here a large difference between LCA and RCA can be observed.

Figure 6.23 shows the number of optimisation steps on each resolution level for iteration 3, i.e. with a gating window size of $\omega = 1.0$. For the initial alignment on the lowest resolution level, the top range of values is increased compared to iterations 1 and 2. Registration on levels 2 and 3 behaved similarly, with more steps taken for RCA on both levels. On level 4, the amount of steps needed is lower for those projections with previous knowledge from iteration 2. On the highest resolution level, this is still visible but less pronounced.

The difference between registration with and without previous knowledge is whether the process starts on level 1 or 4. In both cases, a B-spline motion model with $c = 6$ serves as input to level 4. It is either the previous knowledge or the result

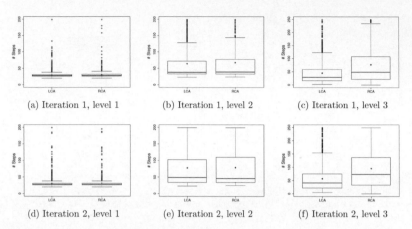

(a) Iteration 1, level 1   (b) Iteration 1, level 2   (c) Iteration 1, level 3

(d) Iteration 2, level 1   (e) Iteration 2, level 2   (f) Iteration 2, level 3

Figure 6.22: Optimisation steps for iterations 1 and 2 ($\omega = 0.4$). On level 1 and 2 M_{affine}, on level 3 M_{spline} with $c = 6$ is estimated (cf. Sec. 3.3).

of level 3. The use of previous knowledge therefore cannot explain the difference in registration steps between Fig. 6.23d and Fig. 6.23e. Figure 6.24 shows those B-spline registrations where optimisation was stopped after reaching the maximum number of steps allowed, instead of convergence, together with their heart phase relative to h_r. A strong peak can be seen between 10 % and 20 %. Since the median of h_r was 0.75, this corresponds to a heart phase between 0.85 and 0.95 in most cases. This phase is reported by [Ache 00] to show the fastest coronary motion during the heart cycle.

In Figure 6.25 the initial NCC value before registration is shown for iteration 1 and 3 (the graph for iteration 2 is almost identical to Figure 6.25a and is thus not repeated). The curve for the LCA datasets shows the highest correlation at h_r and a symmetric decrease with distance. The RCA curve exhibits a strong decrease in correlation for $h(i) > h_r$, especially about 10 % after h_r, which corresponds to the observation in the previous paragraph that projection images between 10 % and 20 % after h_r seem to be the most difficult for RCA datasets. In contrast, the LCA curve decays more slowly for $h(i) > h_r$ compared to $h(i) < h_r$.

In Figure 6.26, the average registration time per level and iteration is shown with respect to the relative heart phase of the projection image. The initial alignment on the first level of iteration 1 (Fig. 6.26a) does not show any obvious dependency on either heart phase or LCA/RCA. On the second level (Fig. 6.26b), a moderate dependency on heart phase can be observed. The curves for level 1 and 2 of iteration 2 are almost identical, and are therefore not depicted. On level 3 of iteration 1 (Fig. 6.26c), a clear dependency on heart phase and an increased registration time for RCA are visible. Both LCA and RCA show a steeper increase in registration time for $h(i) > h_r$ compared to $h(i) < h_r$, although the increase is stronger for RCA. In iteration 2, a similar shape of the curves can be seen on level 3 (Fig. 6.26d), but average registration time is increased by 20 %. For LCA, this is mainly due to a

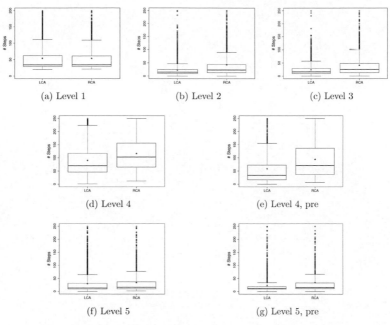

(a) Level 1   (b) Level 2   (c) Level 3

(d) Level 4   (e) Level 4, pre

(f) Level 5   (g) Level 5, pre

Figure 6.23: Optimisation steps for iteration 3 ($\omega = 1.0$). On level 1 M_{affine}, on level 2 and 3 M_{spline} with $c = 6$, and on level 4 and 5 M_{spline} with $c = 12$ is estimated (cf. Sec. 3.3). Pre indicates those registrations where previous knowledge from iteration 2 was used.

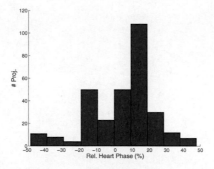

Figure 6.24. B-spline registrations where optimisation was stopped after 250 steps instead of convergence.

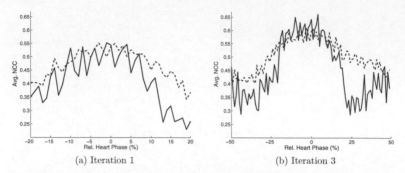

Figure 6.25: Initial NCC value by heart phase relative to h_r. -- LCA, - RCA.

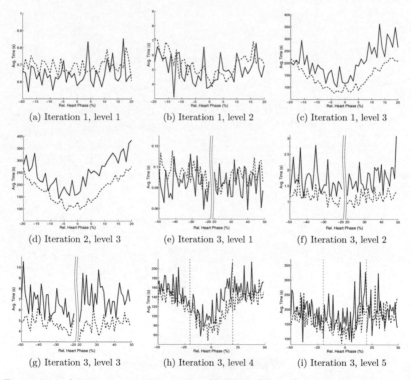

Figure 6.26: Average registration runtime by heart phase relative to h_r.
-- LCA, - RCA. Iteration 1 / 2: On level 1 and 2 M_{affine}, on level 3 M_{spline} with $c = 6$ is estimated. Iteration 3: On level 1 M_{affine}, on level 2 and 3 M_{spline} with $c = 6$ and on level 4 and 5 M_{spline} with $c = 12$ is estimated (cf. Sec. 3.3).

Table 6.9: Average registration times in seconds per projection and iteration. Pre indicates registration with previous knowledge from iteration 2.

Iteration	LCA	RCA
1	147±127	211+180
2	178±137	254±179
3	324±277	353±280
3 (pre)	240±271	306±287

stronger increase in registration time for projections further away from h_r. The time around h_r is almost identical between iteration 1 and 2. On level 1 of iteration 3 (Fig. 6.26e), the runtime behaviour is similar to what was observed for the initial alignment in iteration 1 and 2: No obvious dependency on either heart phase or LCA/RCA. Deformable registration with $c = 6$ (Fig. 6.26f and 6.26g) also does not show a strong dependency on heart phase, but increased registration time for RCA. The first level of deformable registration with $c = 12$ (Fig. 6.26h) shows a strong dependency on heart phase and an increased time for RCA. The transition between registrations with and without previous knowledge (as indicated by the dashed vertical lines) is very smooth. Finally, the highest level of iteration 3 (Fig. 6.26i) displays a weaker dependency on heart phase, with a stronger increase for $h(i) > h_r$, and slightly increased time for RCA. A summary of average total registration times per projection and iteration is listed in Table 6.9.

With the observations of the previous paragraph in mind, the largest contribution to registration time per iteration came from deformable registration. In particular, level 3 of iteration 1 and 2 and level 4 and 5 of iteration 3 had the highest impact on total registration time. Thus, in Figure 6.27 the convergence behaviour of those registrations is depicted for a random selection of 10 % of all projection images. As expected from Figure 6.22 and 6.23, the majority of projection images reached convergence within 150 optimisation steps. For those images, where convergence was reached later or not at all (250 steps), the decrease of $-$NCC was very slow after 150 steps.

In Table 6.10, the runtimes of all components of RMC and NOPMEC in seconds and relative to the total runtime are listed. Since NOPMEC does not do any pre-processing besides what is needed for the regular reconstruction pipeline, the 60 s difference to RMC is the time needed for the pre-processing introduced in Section 3.1.1. Initial reconstruction time is negligible for both algorithms. The time needed for forward projection and bounding box detection is also minor compared to the total runtime of RMC. For both algorithms, about 90 % of the runtime is spent during motion estimation. The total runtime difference between both algorithms is by a factor of 10.

6.4 Discussion and Conclusions

In this chapter, the first part of a human clinical study, the quantitative evaluation of RMC, was presented. To support the evaluation, a software called CoroEval was introduced. It runs on multiple operating systems and is designed to be independent

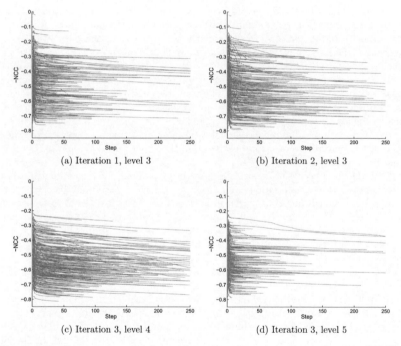

Figure 6.27: Convergence of deformable registration. A random selection of 10 % of all projection images is shown.

Table 6.10: Runtime of RMC and NOPMEC. Missing time between component sum and total is spent in the reconstruction software framework.

	RMC (s)	(%)	NOPMEC (s)	(%)
Pre-proc.	73.5±2.3	1.6	9.5±1.1	2.1
Initial reco.	4.9±1.4	0.1	5.6±1.5	1.2
FwP		0.3		
$\omega = 0.4$ (2×)	2.7±0.6			
$\omega = 1.0$	6.3±1.4			
Bounding box (2×)	4.6±0.1	0.2		
Motion est.		89.8	438.2±99.6	91.5
Iter. 1	752.6±240.1			
Iter. 2	873.9±254.6			
Iter. 3	2843.9±1238.6			
Reconstruction		7.5	18.8±5.1	3.9
$\omega = 0.4$ (2×)	79.2±8.2			
$\omega = 1.0$	177.9±8.9			
Total	4928.6±1491.1		478.8±107.7	

of the imaging modality used. So far, it has been successfully tested on C-arm CT, CT and MRI data. At this point, its purpose is the comparison of reconstruction algorithms or acquisition protocols, not the clinical diagnosis. Implemented metrics are vessel sharpness and diameter. The latter allows for a comparison to reference diameters, which might be available from 2-D QCA data. All measurements are taken from the raw intensity data to be independent of display windows. With default settings, measurements are taken at 1 mm intervals along the vessel centreline and from 10 different angles at each measurement point. This allows for outlier detection and noise-robust measurements without the burden and subjectivity a manual measurement process would incur. We evaluated the diameter measurement process using three phantom datasets, using 2-D QCA on X-ray fluoroscopy data as a reference. An average deviation of 0.03 ± 0.03 mm was found and demonstrates the viability of the software.

58 patient datasets from two clinical sites were available for the study. This allows for a robust and statistically meaningful evaluation. When interpreting the results of sub-groups, the limited amount of measurements in the RCA (19), heart rate (18/18/22) and heart rate variability (50 vs. 8) groups compared to the others has to be considered. Decision on the reference heart phase h_r for each dataset was made by visual comparison of $h_r = 0.75$ and an automatically determined h_r. The results confirmed observations from previous work, that reconstruction at $h_r = 0.75$ is a good choice for the majority of datasets. Five reconstructions (*Initial*, RMC 40 %, RMC 80 %, RMC 100 %, and NOPMEC) were generated from every dataset. The *Initial* volume was used as the reference volume for RMC 40 % and NOPMEC. A common voxel size of 0.5 mm was used for every reconstruction to enable comparison across datasets. For evaluation with CoroEval, a 3-D centreline segmentation of a vessel branch is needed. We segmented the main branch of the LAD and LCX

for every LCA dataset, and the main branch of every RCA dataset. Only those datasets were used for the quantitative evaluation where segmentation was possible for all 5 reconstructions. This resulted in ~80 % of the datasets being used. For 8 of the remaining 19 vessel branches, segmentation of RMC 80 % and RMC 100 % was possible although segmentation of *Initial* and for some even RMC 40 % was not. This means that a segmentation-based motion estimation technique would have failed for these datasets, whereas they could be compensated with RMC. Only one RCA dataset could not be segmented at all, the failure reason of the segmentation algorithm remaining unknown. For the LCA datasets where no segmentation was possible, contrast flow problems can be seen in the acquisitions. Regarding the length of the segmented centreline, which gives an indication of the algorithm performance for small vessels, NOPMEC represented the average length for each dataset. *Initial* resulted in significantly below-average, the RMC variants in significantly above-average lengths.

The sharpness evaluation showed that RMC 80 % resulted in the significantly sharpest vessels. Over all datasets, RMC 100 % was significantly sharper than RMC 40 %. In [Schw 13a] it was shown on six datasets that an increase in the gating window size generally resulted in a decrease in sharpness when the same ramp filter kernel was used. The decrease could be more than compensated by using a sharper kernel for $\omega \geq 0.8$. This experiment was not repeated in the larger clinical study here, but its conclusions can be safely transferred to this study: Reconstructions with a normal kernel and $\omega \geq 0.8$ were also always sharper here than those with a smooth kernel and $\omega = 0.4$. Datasets in the low heart rate group generally resulted in the sharpest reconstructions. Between the medium and high heart rate groups, the sharpness of *Initial*, RMC 40 % and NOPMEC was largely unchanged, while the sharpness of RMC 80 % and RMC 100 % increased again. Since heart rate influences e.g. the number of projection images per heart cycle, movement speed and length of rest phases, a combination of different effects seems to interact here, which is not yet well understood. Since not many datasets with a high heart rate variability were available, no strong conclusions on its influence can be made. From the available data, low variability resulted in sharper vessels, although the influence was not as high as for heart rate. Practical experience from CT imaging seems to suggest the contrary, i.e. heart rate variability having a higher influence on reconstruction quality than heart rate. Therefore, no definite conclusions on this aspect can be gained from the available data in this study.

Vessel diameter evaluation could be performed for ~66 % of all datasets, since in addition to the 3-D segmentations for CoroEval, suitable acquisitions for 2-D QCA need to be available. The standard deviation of repeated 2-D QCA measurements was 0.14 mm. The majority of all reconstructions over all datasets showed a deviation of less than 0.5 mm from the 2-D reference. *Initial* resulted in systematically too large vessels. All RMC variants underestimated vessel sizes to different degrees. NOPMEC systematically overestimated vessel sizes. RMC 100 % and NOPMEC had the lowest deviations, both on average within the estimated accuracy of the 2-D reference. A high heart rate and/or variability increases the diameter error of *Initial*, while the effect on the RMC variants is minimal. NOPMEC is affected most in the high heart rate group.

The runtime evaluation of RMC showed a large difference between LCA and RCA datasets. On level 3 of iteration 1 and 2, deformable registration of the RCA datasets needed twice as many optimisation steps as for the LCA datasets. This is supported by the faster decrease in initial NCC of the RCA datasets for $h(i) \neq h_r$ (especially $h(i) > h_r$), which indicates more registration effort. Overall, 96–98 % of the registration time was spent on levels with M_{spline}, while the registration time itself was responsible for ~90 % of the total algorithm runtime. When looking at iteration 3, where M_{spline} is estimated on multiple resolution levels with varying c, most time is spent on the highest level. This confirms the analysis from Section 3.2, that the number of pixels in a projection image (which changes with resolution level) has the most influence on algorithm runtime. In [Schw 13b], it was shown that an average ROI size of 36 % of the image size resulted in a runtime reduction of 41 % (LCA) and 24 % (RCA). This experiment was not repeated for the larger clinical study, but since the average ROI size was also 36 % here, a similar relation may be expected. A further reduction of the ROI size by calculating individual ROIs for every projection image could possibly lead to a further speedup, but a balance with algorithm stability needs to be found here. Using the union of all individual ROIs helps to avoid misdetected ROIs.

Another optimisation potential, where further evaluation is needed before final conclusions can be drawn, is the maximum allowed number of optimisation steps. In the study, the majority of deformable registrations converged in less than 150 steps, while the remaining showed a very slow improvement. Whether a maximum of 150 instead of 250 can help in improving registration time without sacrificing image quality needs to be carefully examined.

When comparing the registration time per projection (Table 6.9) times the number of projections (~50 for iterations 1 and 2, 133 for iteration 3) with the average time per iteration (Table 6.10), a difference of a factor of 10 is obvious. This comes from the multi-processing effect of running 16 registration processes in parallel. Therefore, registration time can also highly benefit from modern many-CPU architectures. Still, RMC uses non-optimised CPU code from ITK (cf. Sec. 3.1.4) for registration. NOPMEC uses a highly optimised B-spline motion model integrated into the reconstruction algorithm on the graphics card [Rohk 10b, Rohk 11]. This is the main contributing factor to the high runtime difference between NOPMEC and RMC, which makes the interventional use of RMC difficult at this time. But an adaption of the motion model and NCC evaluation onto the graphics card promises a strong reduction in registration time, since parallel processing can be exploited to an even higher degree on the graphics card.

Finally, both quantitative and runtime measurements showed that RCA datasets seem to be more difficult than LCA, which is consistent with similar findings for CT-based coronary angiography [Ache 00, Niem 01]. RCA datasets consistently resulted in worse sharpness (especially *Initial*, which influences registration effort), worse initial NCC for $h(i) \neq h_r$ and longer runtimes. Especially for the RCA datasets, projection images between 10 % and 20 % after h_r showed the highest effort and worst initial NCC. These projection images are from a phase where fast heart motion occurs [Ache 00], which can lead to motion blur even within the acquired X-ray projections due to the limited detector frame rate. Obviously, such errors in the acquired data cannot be corrected by a motion compensation algorithm and pose an additional difficulty during motion estimation. Other possible influencing factors on the difference between left and right coronary arteries could be their three-dimensional shape and actual motion patterns (as opposed to just the speed of motion). Both these factors were not further investigated in this study.

It could be shown that RMC can be successfully applied to a large set of clinical data without adjustment of parameters and with a high robustness against the quality of the initial reconstruction: Over the various sub-groups, the quality metrics for the initial reconstructions vary considerably, while the effect on the RMC-compensated reconstructions is distinctly lower. RMC 80 % and RMC 100 % consistently outperformed *Initial*, RMC 40 % and NOPMEC, with RMC 80 % resulting in sharper vessels and RMC 100 % in less diameter error.

Human Clinical Study – Qualitative Evaluation

In this chapter, the qualitative evaluation of the human clinical study introduced in the last chapter is presented. A non-blinded observer study with one anatomically trained observer was performed. In the previous chapter, only the three main branches of the coronary tree were analysed. They are both the clinically most relevant vessels, as well as allow for the reliable centreline extraction necessary for the quantitative analysis. In this chapter, also smaller vessels and side branches are investigated. This is to evaluate the visual impression of the reconstructions, which for a human observer will be influenced by the whole picture that is seen. On the other hand, it is clear that those smaller vessels represent a much harder problem for reconstruction algorithms.

In Section 7.1, the rating process and further analysis are described. The results of the observer study are presented in Section 7.2. Example images for 4 LCA and 4 RCA datasets are shown in Section 7.3. A discussion concludes this chapter.

Parts of this chapter have been published in [Schw 14b].

7.1 Rating and Analysis

All 58 patient datasets were subject to qualitative evaluation by one observer. The observer was not blinded regarding the algorithm and parameters of an image. Since one patient had a total occlusion of the LAD, 38 LAD, 39 LCX and 19 RCA were evaluated segment-wise. Each segment of each reconstruction of each dataset was rated individually on a scale of 0 to 3:

- 0: Not visible at all.

- 1: Visible, but corrupted by artefacts.

- 2: Acceptable to good quality.

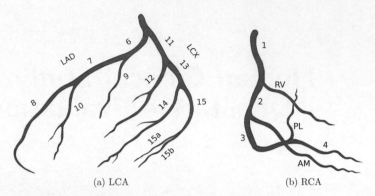

(a) LCA   (b) RCA

Figure 7.1: Vessel segments used for qualitative evaluation.
Original images[1] © Patrick J. Lynch, medical illustrator; C. Carl Jaffe, MD, cardiologist.
Modified and used under `http://creativecommons.org/licenses/by/2.5`.

- 3: Perfect quality.

Figure 7.1 shows an illustration of the segments that were used for evaluation. The segments follow the 15 segment model coronary artery classification system [Aust 75], with the addition of several small vessel segments. These smaller segments were not assigned unique identifiers in the original classification, but clearly identifiable in many reconstructions and therefore included here. On the other hand, segment 5, the communal main branch of the left coronary artery, was not included in this evaluation. Owing to the acquisition protocol, this section generally cannot be reconstructed due to the direct strong contrast inflow at this position. The 19 numbered segments correspond to the following anatomical features:

- LAD: proximal (6), medial (7) and distal/apical (8) main branch. First (9) and second (10) diagonal branch.

- LCX: proximal (11), medial (13) and distal (15) main branch. Obtuse marginal (12), postero-lateral (14, 15a) and atrioventricular (15b) branches.

- RCA: proximal (1), medial (2) and distal (3) main branch. Right-ventricular (RV), acute marginal (AM), posterior descending (4) and postero-lateral (PL) branches.

If the individual patient anatomy displayed more or less side branches than described here, care was taken by the observer to always rate the same side branches for all 5 reconstructions of that dataset. Missing branches were handled in the analysis of the rating results. If all five ratings for one vessel segment were 0, the segment was assumed missing in the original data and not considered for the evaluation of this dataset.

---

[1]`http://commons.wikimedia.org/wiki/File:Heart_left_lateral_diagrams.svg`, `http://commons.wikimedia.org/wiki/File:Heart_right_anterior_oblique_diagrams.svg`

Table 7.1: Vessel segment groups for small and large vessels.

	Small	Large
LAD	8, 9, 10	6, 7
LCX	12, 14, 15, 15a, 15b	11, 13
RCA	3, 4, RV, AM, PL	1, 2

From these individual segment ratings, one overall score for each reconstruction was calculated by taking the mean rating over all segments where at least one reconstruction had a rating larger than zero. In addition, two more scores were calculated to reflect the reconstruction quality of small and large vessels. For these scores, the mean rating was calculated over the two groups of segments listed in Table 7.1, again excluding segments where all reconstructions were rated 0. Finally, datasets were grouped by heart rate and heart rate variability in the same way as in the previous chapter.

Statistical analysis of the results was performed in the same way as laid out in Section 6.2.3. Due to large between-datasets variation of the ratings, the score distributions for each reconstruction type were not normally distributed. Since only the difference of two distributions needs to be normally distributed for a paired t-test, we show the pairwise difference distributions in Q–Q plots.

7.2   Results

Figure 7.2 shows the results of the overall observer ratings. There is a clear trend for RMC 100 % reconstructions to receive the highest ratings. Only in the RCA group (Fig. 7.2d) are the distributions of RMC 80 % and RMC 100 % very close together. Regarding vessel type, LCX and RCA received slightly higher ratings than LAD. The distributions of the ratings of the NOPMEC reconstructions were very similar to those of the RMC 40 % reconstructions, with the exception of the RCA. NOPMEC also had the highest spread of scores. As expected, *Initial* constantly received the lowest ratings, with little difference between vessel types. What is common for all reconstructions is that the median scores are all below 2, meaning the typical overall score was less than "acceptable to good quality". Although the whiskers extend to 3, this demands a more fine-grained examination than the overall score can achieve. Therefore, further in this section, sub-groups are examined for a better understanding of the data.

Figure 7.3 shows the Q–Q plots for the overall observer ratings. All distributions display reasonable similarity to a normal distribution. Table 7.2 lists the results of the t-tests. The observation of the distributions of RMC 40 % and NOPMEC being similar (with the exception of RCA) is confirmed here. Also for RCA, RMC 80 % and RMC 100 % do not show a significant difference in their ratings, as suspected above.

Since the overall rating is the average score over all vessel segments, it might be influenced by poor ratings of small vessels. We therefore also calculated average ratings over groups of segments. Figure 7.4 shows the results of the observer ratings for large vessels. Here, the median scores are distinctly higher than for the overall ratings. RMC 100 % still is the highest rated reconstruction type, with a large overlap

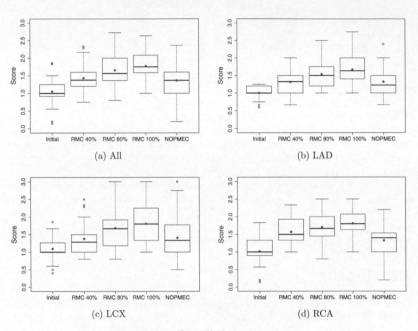

Figure 7.2: Overall observer ratings.

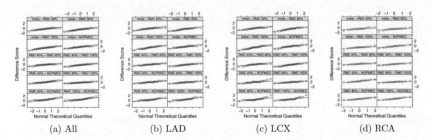

Figure 7.3: Q–Q plots of the distributions of overall observer ratings.

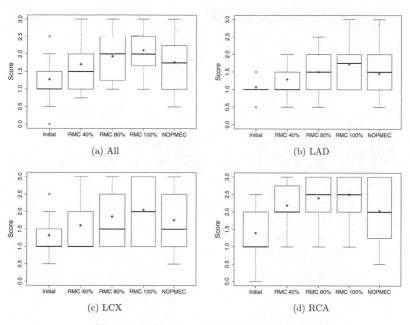

Figure 7.4: Observer ratings for large vessels.

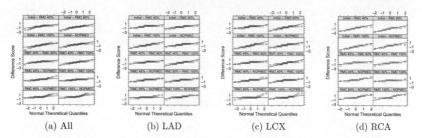

Figure 7.5: Q–Q plots of the distributions of observer ratings for large vessels.

Table 7.2: Significance of differences in overall observer ratings.

(a) All

	Initial	40%	80%	100%
40%	★★★			
80%	★★★	★★★		
100%	★★★	★★★	★★★	
NOPMEC	★★★	○	★★★	★★★

(b) LAD

	Initial	40%	80%	100%
40%	★★★			
80%	★★★	★★★		
100%	★★★	★★★	★	
NOPMEC	★★★	○	★★	★★★

(c) LCX

	Initial	40%	80%	100%
40%	★★★			
80%	★★★	★★★		
100%	★★★	★★★	★★	
NOPMEC	★★★	○	★★	★★★

(d) RCA

	Initial	40%	80%	100%
40%	★★★			
80%	★★★	★		
100%	★★★	★★	○	
NOPMEC	★★	★	★★★	★★★

with RMC 80% and NOPMEC. Especially for RCA, all compensated reconstruction types were rated very similarly and high.

Figure 7.5 shows the Q–Q plots for the observer ratings for large vessels. Most distributions display reasonable similarity to a normal distribution. But especially the RMC 40%–NOPMEC, RMC 80%–NOPMEC and RMC 100%–NOPMEC pairs deviate from normal distributions in the upper tail. Table 7.3 lists the results of the t-tests. The observations from above regarding the large overlap of distributions for RCA are confirmed.

Table 7.3: Significance of differences in observer ratings for large vessels.

(a) All

	Initial	40%	80%	100%
40%	★★★			
80%	★★★	★★★		
100%	★★★	★★★	★★★	
NOPMEC	★★★	○	○	★★★

(b) LAD

	Initial	40%	80%	100%
40%	★★			
80%	★★★	★★		
100%	★★★	★★★	★★	
NOPMEC	★★★	○	○	★★

(c) LCX

	Initial	40%	80%	100%
40%	★★			
80%	★★★	★★★		
100%	★★★	★★★	★	
NOPMEC	★★★	○	○	★

(d) RCA

	Initial	40%	80%	100%
40%	★★★			
80%	★★★	○		
100%	★★★	○	○	
NOPMEC	★★	○	○	○

Figure 7.6 shows the results of the observer ratings for small vessels. It is clear that the small vessels are the reason for the lower overall ratings observed. Here, RMC 80% and RMC 100% are very close together. For RCA, all maximum ratings are distinctly lower than for the other vessel types. In comparison with the large

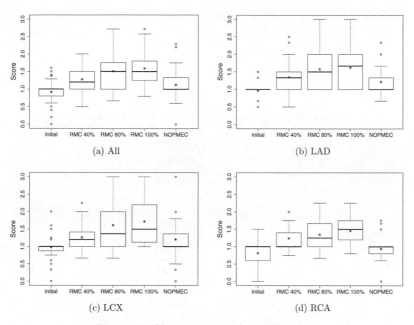

(a) All

(b) LAD

(c) LCX

(d) RCA

Figure 7.6: Observer ratings for small vessels.

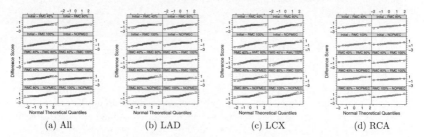

(a) All

(b) LAD

(c) LCX

(d) RCA

Figure 7.7: Q–Q plots of the distributions of observer ratings for small vessels.

vessel group, NOPMEC scored lower than the RMC variants, more similar to *Initial* than RMC 40 % here.

Figure 7.7 shows the Q–Q plots for the observer ratings for small vessels. All distributions display reasonable similarity to a normal distribution. Table 7.4 lists the results of the *t*-tests. The observation of the overlap between RMC 80 % and RMC 100 % is confirmed here. For RCA, no significant difference could be found for the RMC 40 % –RMC 80 %, RMC 40 % –RMC 100 % and RMC 40 % –NOPMEC pairs.

Table 7.4: Significance of differences in observer ratings for small vessels.

(a) All

	Initial	40 %	80 %	100 %
40 %	★★★			
80 %	★★★	★★★		
100 %	★★★	★★★	★	
NOPMEC	★★★	★	★★★	★★★

(b) LAD

	Initial	40 %	80 %	100 %
40 %	★★★			
80 %	★★★	★★		
100 %	★★★	★★★	○	
NOPMEC	★★	○	★★	★★★

(c) LCX

	Initial	40 %	80 %	100 %
40 %	★★★			
80 %	★★★	★★★		
100 %	★★★	★★★	○	
NOPMEC	○	○	★★★	★★★

(d) RCA

	Initial	40 %	80 %	100 %
40 %	★★			
80 %	★★★	○		
100 %	★★★	○	○	
NOPMEC	○	○	★★	★★★

Figure 7.8 shows the results of the observer ratings grouped by heart rate. The relative relation between reconstruction types is the same over all three groups. Neither the RMC variants nor NOPMEC show a large influence of heart rate on the observer ratings. *Initial* is affected most, with a small decrease in score as heart rate increases.

Figure 7.9 shows the Q–Q plots for the observer ratings grouped by heart rate. All distributions display reasonable similarity to a normal distribution. Table 7.5 lists the results of the *t*-tests.

Figure 7.10 shows the results of the observer ratings grouped by heart rate variability. Scores are slightly lower in the high HRV group, with the most effect on *Initial* and NOPMEC.

7.3   Image Examples

Four LCA and four RCA datasets were selected to display both variety in anatomy as well as different quality of the initial reconstruction. They are shown in Figure 7.12 and 7.13. Since all reconstruction variants result in different HU values of the reconstructed vessels, the greyscale window centre was determined automatically and individually for each reconstructed volume for a fair comparison. The same procedure as outlined in Section 3.1.3 was used to find a window centre such that only the t_r percentile of the largest voxel values is visible. A threshold of $t_r = 0.5 \%$ (LCA) and $t_r = 0.3 \%$ (RCA) was used. The window width was 1000 HU for reconstructions with $\omega = 0.4$. For the other reconstructions, the window width was 2000 HU (LCA) and

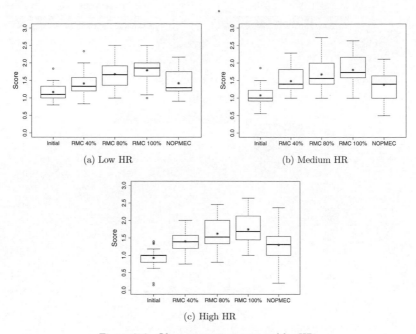

(a) Low HR

(b) Medium HR

(c) High HR

Figure 7.8: Observer ratings grouped by HR.

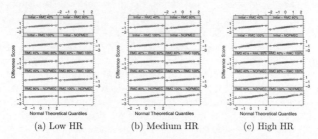

(a) Low HR   (b) Medium HR   (c) High HR

Figure 7.9: Q–Q plots of the distributions of observer ratings grouped by HR.

Table 7.5: Significance of differences in observer ratings grouped by HR.

(a) Low HR

	Initial	40%	80%	100%
40%	★			
80%	★★★	★★★		
100%	★★★	★★★	○	
NOPMEC	★	○	★★★	★★★

(b) Medium HR

	Initial	40%	80%	100%
40%	★★★			
80%	★★★	★		
100%	★★★	★★★	○	
NOPMEC	★★	○	○	★★

(c) High HR

	Initial	40%	80%	100%
40%	★★★			
80%	★★★	★★		
100%	★★★	★★★	★	
NOPMEC	★★★	○	★★	★★

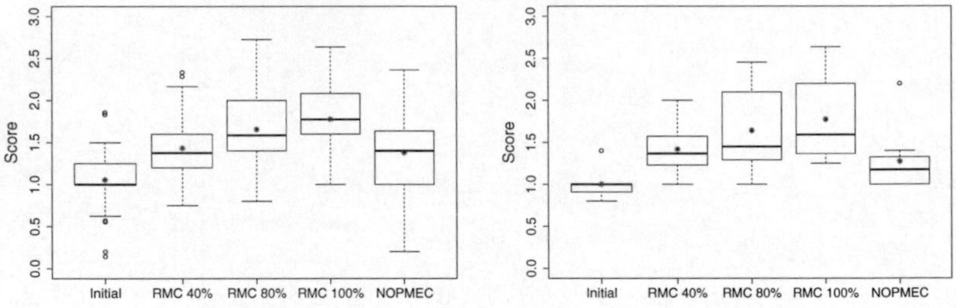

(a) Low HRV   (b) High HRV

Figure 7.10: Observer ratings grouped by HRV.

3000 HU (RCA). By this procedure, the different contrast and intensity behaviours of the algorithms are taken into account. Thus, the influence of these factors on vessel visibility and thus observer rating is minimised.

The benefit of using more data and a sharper filter kernel is clearly visible when comparing RMC 40% with RMC 80% and RMC 100%. Also, the recovery of structure even for datasets with bad initial quality is demonstrated (e.g. the second LCA). Between RMC 80% and RMC 100%, the most distal parts of the vessels became less visible. On the other hand, the artefact level decreased and vessel homogeneity increased at RMC 100%, which correlates with this variant receiving higher ratings than RMC 80%. Figure 7.11 shows a magnified detail of the artificial aortic valve of the fourth LCA. Here, the benefit of using more data is emphasised again by the visibility of fine-detailed structure.

The observations of Section 7.2 regarding NOPMEC can be confirmed in these example images: Display of distal vessels is comparable with RMC 40%, for small vessels with *Initial*. Performance for RCA is worse than for LCA.

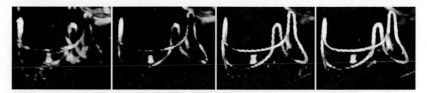

Figure 7.11: Magnified detail of LCA 4. From left to right: *Initial*, RMC 40 %, RMC 80 % and RMC 100 %.

7.4   Discussion and Conclusions

In this chapter, the second part of the human clinical study, the qualitative evaluation of RMC, was presented. All 58 datasets, including those with contrast problems (cf. Section 6.3.1), were evaluated by one human observer. The observer rated individual vessel segments of each reconstruction. From these ratings, an overall score per reconstruction was calculated as the mean value of the segment ratings. In addition, scores for small and large vessels, as well as ratings grouped by heart rate and heart rate variability were calculated.

Although the results of the overall dataset ratings suggest a median rating of less than 2 ("acceptable to good quality") for all reconstruction types, it has to be kept in mind that this includes at least 12 datasets of very bad quality, which were not part of the evaluation in the previous chapter due to non-existing centrelines. Also, very small distal vessels are included, where motion estimation is more difficult. The cost functions of the evaluated motion estimation algorithms are influenced more by larger vessels than smaller ones, simply due to their averaging nature over a whole image or volume. In addition, small vessels display less contrast due to less contrast agent accumulation compared to a larger vessel.

When only the larger vessels are considered in calculating a dataset rating, the results look much more promising: The median score for RMC 80 % and RMC 100 % was 2 over all datasets, with RMC 100 % being the highest rated reconstruction type. This is an important result, since proximal and medial segments are the most important sites for percutaneous coronary interventions. Those parts of the coronary arteries feed the largest portion of the myocardial mass and stenosis there would incur the greatest damage. Therefore, stenosis in distal vessels is usually not treated, whereas a clear depiction of the proximal and medial parts is clinically very relevant.

Examination of the scores for small vessels confirmed that the overall scores are indeed highly influenced by these ratings. Since the average overall score per dataset was calculated over 2 large and 3 (LAD) or 5 (LCX/RCA) small vessel segments (cf. Table 7.1), the low ratings of these segments reduce the overall quality scores. Still, all RMC variants showed significant improvement of vessel quality over *Initial*. Interestingly, while the top range of scores reached 3 for LAD and LCX, it is greatly reduced for RCA, which is not the case in the large vessel group. This lower quality for smaller segments might be another correlation with the higher effort for RCA datasets observed in the previous chapter. Looking at the ratings for NOPMEC, significantly lower scores in the small vessel group were observed (compared to RMC 80 % and RMC

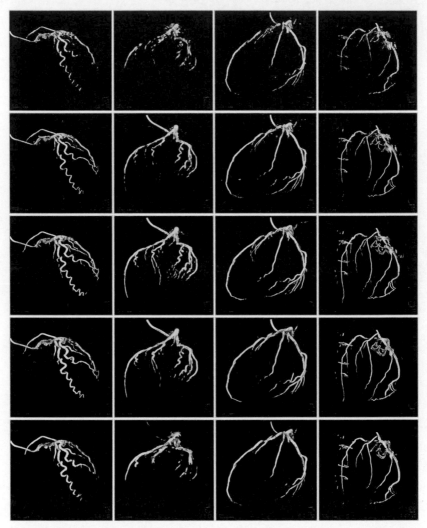

Figure 7.12: Left coronary arteries. From top to bottom: *Initial*, RMC 40 %, RMC 80 %, RMC 100 %, NOPMEC. From left to right: Datasets LCA1–4.

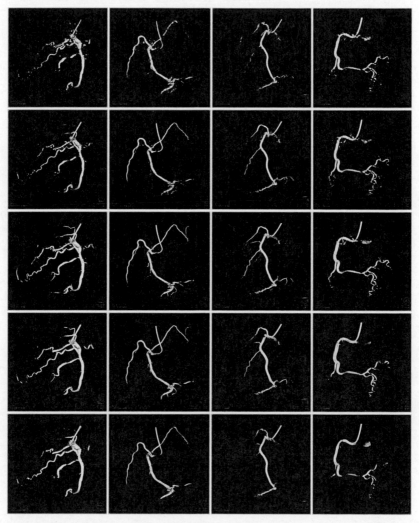

Figure 7.13: Right coronary arteries. From top to bottom: *Initial*, RMC 40 %, RMC 80 %, RMC 100 %, NOPMEC. From left to right: Datasets RCA1–4.

100 %). This is the most probable reason for its overall scores being significantly lower, too, comparable to RMC 40 %.

Regarding the influence of heart rate and heart rate variability, no large influence of either on the RMC-compensated reconstructions could be found. The observation from the previous chapter, that RMC reconstructions are relatively robust against the quality of the initial reconstruction, could be further confirmed here. *Initial* was affected a lot more by increasing heart rate than the RMC-compensated reconstructions. NOPMEC was affected by heart rate variability. It makes use of a time-continuous B-spline for temporal modelling, while RMC has one 2-D motion field for every time point. This might be an indication that a high temporal resolution (i.e. full sampling like RMC or more temporal control points) is necessary to capture heart rate variations.

Comparing the findings of this chapter to the quantitative evaluation, a good correlation can be found. Although RMC 80 % always had sharper vessels than RMC 100 %, the observer consistently rated RMC 100 % higher. When looking at the example images, it can be seen that the observer weighted artefact-free vessels higher than a slight reduction in sharpness. Since RMC 100 % also resulted in less diameter error, a preference towards $\omega = 1.0$ can be stated.

RCA datasets were observed to take longer for motion estimation and result in less sharp vessels in the previous chapter. Here, their median ratings were not worse than for the LCA datasets (for the RMC variants). This is an encouraging result. It means that although they seem to pose more difficulty for motion estimation, the subjective quality of RMC-compensated reconstructions of RCA is equivalent to LCA to the human observer in this study.

CHAPTER 8

Summary and Outlook

8.1 Summary

Cardiovascular disease is the number one cause of death worldwide. Its prevention, diagnosis and therapy are therefore very important topics in today's medicine. Especially for diagnosis, and even more so therapy, fluoroscopy-guided interventions in the catheter laboratory have become a method of choice. The C-arm systems used for these interventions allow for a large freedom in positioning the X-ray source and detector with respect to the patient. Still, the angiographic images they produce are two-dimensional and as such limited in the depiction of complex spatial relations. Today this is alleviated by acquiring projections from several angles and physicians assembling the information in their head. On the other hand, a C-arm system is capable of rotating around the patient on a circular trajectory with enough angular coverage to facilitate a CT-like 3-D reconstruction. The major problem encountered there is the slow rotation speed of the system. In a typical rotation of 3–5 seconds, the object of interest – the heart – beats several times. This means that a direct reconstruction of the 3-D image leads to a result that is heavily degraded by motion artefacts. Therefore there is a need for motion estimation and compensation algorithms to enable CT-like interventional imaging of cardiovascular structures like the coronary arteries. This was the topic of this thesis: To develop and study the properties of such a motion estimation and compensation algorithm for coronary arteries.

In Chapter 2, the state of the art was discussed. Generally speaking, methods can be distinguished into model-based and tomographic reconstructions. The former result in a centreline and/or lumen model, the latter in a tomographic image. Most of the existing model-based methods either require manual interaction, which is not desirable in an interventional setting, or a reliable 2-D centreline extraction, which is a difficult and so far unsolved task for clinical data. On the other hand, they can work with non-well-calibrated systems and require much less projection images than tomographic methods. Straight-forward tomographic reconstruction methods cannot be applied to cardiac C-arm CT data, for the reasons already discussed. If a periodic heart motion is assumed, an ECG-gated reconstruction can be performed. This can serve as a good initial estimate for further approaches, but in itself does not satisfy image quality expectations due to undersampling artefacts. More complex motion compensation methods can be categorised by the dimensionality of their motion model. The choice of a 3-D motion model seems natural, but leads to a high-dimensional optimisation problem. The approaches found in the literature use either periodicity assumptions or strong regularisation to alleviate this. The state-of-the-art

NOPMEC algorithm that is also introduced in detail in Chapter 2 uses a simple cost function and integrates the motion estimation into a highly optimised reconstruction algorithm to be able to work with a 3-D motion model. 2-D–3-D registration-based methods, where a 3-D motion model is estimated from 2-D–3-D-correspondences, also suffer from high computational complexity and an ill-conditioned optimisation problem. The algorithms found in the literature make use of easily detectable markers in the projection images or simplified, non-deformable motion models. 2-D motion estimation approaches are limited by the lack of depth information for a given projection, but are attractive due to their reduced computational complexity and reduced ill-posedness. There is also evidence both in the literature and in this thesis, that the missing depth information is not a severe limitation for coronary artery motion. What is missing from the state of the art as found in literature, is an algorithm that neither requires user interaction, nor markers, nor any explicit vessel segmentation, and does not assume a strictly periodic heart motion.

Chapter 3 introduced RMC, a method for projection-based motion estimation using 2-D–2-D image registration. This is the algorithmic contribution of this work. It does not require any user interaction or complex segmentation methods and is fully automatic. The method is embedded in an iterative algorithm that performs motion estimation and compensation in alternation, until a previously defined target is reached (either maximum number of steps or minimal gradient magnitude). An ECG-gated reconstruction serves as the initial input into the first iteration. Since the gating window size in ECG-gating is a trade-off between undersampling and motion-related artefacts, the gating window size is increased from iteration to iteration in a bootstrapping process, until all of the acquired projection data is used for reconstruction of the 3-D image. In addition, a streak reduction method is employed to improve the image quality of the ECG-gated reconstructions. To stabilise and speed up the registration process, several methods are employed. First, the registration is embedded in a multi-resolution scheme. Both the flexibility of the motion model as well as the depth of the multi-resolution scheme are increased between iterations to make use of increasing image quality. Second, a copy of the projection images is pre-processed with morphological operations and thresholding to remove as many non-vascular structures as possible. At the same time, the intermediate 3-D reconstructions are also thresholded to retain only high intensity structures. Third, after forward projection of these thresholded volumes, an automatic region of interest detection algorithm defines the area where the registration process shall take place. This was shown to drastically improve the performance of the registration. Since the grey values in the processed projection images and the maximum intensity forward-projected images differ, the objective function of the registration algorithm has to be able to handle this. Therefore normalised cross-correlation is employed in RMC, which is insensitive to these grey value differences, while being parameter-free and less computationally intensive than mutual information. A gradient descent optimiser is used to drive the registration process. During motion-compensated image reconstruction, it turns out that application of the 2-D motion model can be realised as a simple coordinate transform that can be integrated into the backprojection operation of a standard FDK-type algorithm. Previous 2-D motion compensation algorithms em-

ployed an image transformation and an unmodified backprojection step, which leads
to unnecessary multiple image interpolations.

In Chapter 4, RMC was evaluated in a simulation study with a numerical phantom.
Two phantom configurations were used, a single sphere or a grid of $5 \times 5 \times 5$ spheres,
both floating in free space. The phantoms were generated both static and in heart
cycle-like motion. Using a trajectory from a real C-arm system, simulated projection images were generated from the phantoms. These were then used as input to
create seven reconstructions, ranging from simple FDK, over pure ECG-gated, three
RMC-based reconstructions with various gating window sizes, to two NOPMEC-based
reconstructions. Normalised cross-correlation, diameter measurements and eccentricity were used as metrics to quantify the reconstruction accuracy. The single sphere
experiments showed an overestimation of the sphere's diameter and a non-spherical
shape for all motion-compensated reconstructions. It seems the dataset presents a
very badly conditioned optimisation problem for both NOPMEC and RMC due to the
possibility of estimating any arbitrary motion in the empty areas without penalising
either cost function. NOPMEC was more affected than RMC due to its lower number of spatial B-spline control points. Looking at the diameter error, even the FDK
reconstruction of the static dataset had an error of 0.4 mm. This can be seen as a
lower bound for the measurement accuracy due to the reconstructed voxel size of
0.56 mm and partial volume effects from the high contrast object. In the sphere grid
experiments, the RMC-based reconstruction using all projection data resulted in the
best correlation and the best in-motion shape measurements, followed by NOPMEC.
This demonstrates the self-regularisation of the motion models when more objects
are present compared to the single sphere experiments. Another important result is
that no practical difference between the two NOPMEC-based variants could be found.
One had all possible degrees of freedom in its motion model, while the other was
restricted to motion perpendicular to the current viewing direction for a given time
point. This means that, for a given time / view point, missing depth information in
the motion model does not affect the results noticeably in the presented experiments.
This strengthens the case for a 2-D-based motion estimation scheme. Finally, this
chapter established approximations for the inherent error of the different investigated algorithms. For the static datasets, all errors can only come from the image
reconstruction. As mentioned above, for the FDK reconstructions, the errors represent the baseline quality of the selected cone-beam reconstruction parameters. For
the motion-compensated reconstructions, the additional errors are introduced by the
respective motion estimation and compensation algorithms.

In Chapter 5, the RMC algorithm was tested using the CAVAREV platform. Several
reconstructions with a different number of iterations and different filter kernel choices
were submitted. Due to the strictly periodic nature of the motion in the CAVAREV
dataset, ECG-gating already performs very well. One key result of the chapter was
on the selection of filter kernels. The small 40 % gating window used in the beginning
of the RMC execution leads to undersampling artefacts in the reconstruction. These
are amplified by a sharper kernel, explaining a lower score of small gating window
and sharp kernel. Therefore, a smooth kernel should be used for both the initial
reconstruction as well as all motion-compensated reconstructions with small gating
window sizes. Increasing the gating window size lead to higher scores due to a better

reconstruction of the vasculature. This could be further improved by a sharper kernel, since undersampling artefacts are not as prominent in the reconstructions with larger gating window sizes. Overall, the RMC-based results were the leading results on the CAVAREV website at the time of publication, having been surpassed by [Taub 17] after four years.

The quantitative evaluation of RMC on human clinical data was presented in Chapter 6. A software called CoroEval was introduced to support this evaluation. The software allows the calculation of vessel sharpness and diameter as quantitative metrics for the comparison of reconstruction algorithms. The study introduced in this chapter was carried out on 58 patient datasets from two clinical sites. Five reconstructions were generated for every dataset: An ECG-gated reconstruction (*Initial*), three RMC-based reconstructions using various gating window sizes (RMC 40 %, RMC 80 % and RMC 100 %), and a NOPMEC-based reconstruction. Quantitative evaluation was only performed on those ~80 % of the datasets where 3-D coronary branch segmentation was possible for all five reconstructions. For 8 out of the remaining (non-segmentable) 19 datasets, segmentation would have been possible in the RMC-based reconstructions using 80 % or 100 % of the projection data. This means a sufficient image quality could be achieved after all RMC iterations, although initial image quality was bad. The length of the segmented centrelines can be taken as an indication for the algorithms' performance in small vessels. *Initial* resulted in the shortest centrelines, NOPMEC in the average length and the RMC reconstructions in the longest centrelines. Regarding the sharpness measure, RMC 80 % resulted in the significantly sharpest vessels, while RMC 100 % was still significantly sharper than RMC 40 %. A low heart rate generally also resulted in the sharpest reconstructions. Vessel diameter evaluation could only be performed on ~66 % of all datasets. Only for these datasets suitable 2-D QCA data was available as a ground truth. The majority of all reconstructions resulted in a deviation of less than 0.5 mm from the reference diameter measurements. The diameter error of *Initial* increased with high heart rate and/or variability, while the RMC variants were largely unaffected. NOPMEC was affected by a high heart rate. A large runtime difference between NOPMEC and RMC was found, which makes interventional use of RMC difficult at this time. This can be attributed to RMC using non-optimised CPU code from ITK for its registration pipeline, while NOPMEC uses a highly optimised B-spline motion model on the graphics card. Section 8.2.1 summarises suggestions on how this bottleneck could possibly be opened in the future. In the runtime evaluation of RMC, a large difference between LCA and RCA datasets was found. Deformable registration needed up to twice as many optimisation steps for RCA datasets than for LCA datasets. Since the registration time was responsible for ~90 % of the total algorithm runtime, this is an important observation. The quantitative evaluation of the reconstruction results also confirmed that RCA datasets seem to be more difficult than LCA datasets. Interestingly, especially for RCA datasets, projection images between 10 % and 20 % after the reference heart phase of 75 % showed the highest effort and worst initial NCC values. Since fast heart motion occurs in these phases, there is the possibility for motion blur in the acquired projection images. A motion compensation algorithm cannot correct these errors in its input projection data. Overall, it could be shown that RMC can be successfully applied to a large set of clinical data without adjustment of parameters and with a high robustness against the quality of the initial reconstruction. RMC 80 % and RMC 100 % consistently outperformed *Initial*, RMC 40 % and NOPMEC. RMC 80 % resulted in sharper vessels and RMC 100 % in less diameter error.

All 58 datasets were also qualitatively evaluated by a human observer. The results of this evaluation were presented in Chapter 7. The observer rated the quality of individual vessel segments for each reconstruction. Out of these, an overall average score was calculated per reconstruction. Ratings were additionally grouped by small and large vessels, as well as heart rate and heart rate variability. Since the overall dataset ratings also included datasets of very bad quality that were excluded in Chapter 6, the median rating over all reconstructions was less than "acceptable to good quality". The overall score also includes very small distal vessels, which again lowers the average ratings. When looking only at the ratings for the larger vessels, the median score of RMC 80 % and RMC 100 % was "acceptable to good quality" over all datasets, with RMC 100 % being the highest rated reconstruction type of all. Since proximal and medial segments are the most important sites for coronary interventions, the quality of these segments is the most important. No large influence of heart rate and heart rate variability could be found on the RMC-compensated reconstructions. This further confirms the observation that RMC is relatively robust against the quality of the initial reconstruction. Comparing the qualitative results to the quantitative evaluation, a good correlation was found. Although RMC 80 % resulted in sharper vessels than RMC 100 %, the observer consistently rated the RMC 100 % results higher. When comparing the visual impression of the reconstructions, it can be concluded that the observer preferred artefact-free vessels over a slightly sharper image impression. Together with the lower diameter error of RMC 100 %, there is an overall preference towards RMC 100 % from both the quantitative and qualitative evaluation. Interestingly, although RCA datasets were shown to be more problematic in the quantitative evaluation, their median observer ratings were not worse than those of the LCA datasets (for the RMC variants). This means that even though RCA datasets seem to be more difficult for motion estimation and compensation, the subjective quality of the corresponding RMC-compensated reconstructions was equivalent for the human observer.

8.2 Outlook

In this thesis, a robust method for motion estimation and compensation of coronary arteries in C-arm computed tomography was presented. Looking forward, there are two aspects with potential for further research. First, there is still room for optimisation of the method to bring the computation time down. And second, there are several future applications that can be served by the results of this work.

8.2.1 Optimisation Potentials

As was shown in Chapter 6, the runtime of RMC depends on the quality of the initial reconstruction. Therefore, a straight-forward approach is to improve that quality, e.g. by an improved artefact suppression technique that was recently introduced in

[Taub 16b]. Another finding in Chapter 6 was the strong dependence of the registration time on the amount of pixels in the projection image. As already suggested there, using the smallest possible ROI for each projection instead of the union of all individual ROIs could improve efficiency, but has to be carefully weighed against the stability offered by taking this union. Tuning other parameters, like the maximum amount of registration iterations, might also offer some optimisation potential.

Overall, the largest gain in performance can be expected by using heavily optimised implementations of the normalised cross-correlation and the B-spline motion model, ideally on a graphics card [Ruij 08, Rohk 11, Maie 12]. The ITK framework used in this work offers great flexibility, but contains largely un-optimised, CPU-based code.

8.2.2   Future Applications

Once a 3-D reconstruction of the coronary artery tree is available, several uses beyond the image itself come to mind. First, if a quantitative evaluation of vessel sizes is the goal, an ideal segmentation on the ground-truth 2-D projection images will always be more exact than on the derived 3-D image. On the other hand, as discussed in this thesis, such a 2-D vessel segmentation is difficult. Therefore, one idea could be to support such a segmentation with the information from the 3-D reconstruction and 2-D motion model that are the result of the RMC algorithm. Initial ideas of such an approach were e.g. presented in [Jand 09b, Poly 12].

On the other hand, it is known that the hemodynamic significance of a stenosis cannot be determined fully from morphological information (i.e. diameter-based stenosis degree) alone [Kern 06, Hamm 11, Mont 13]. This is why, in interventional routine, a measurement of the so-called fractional flow reserve (FFR) has become the gold standard for the functional assessment of a stenosis [Pijl 07]. In short, FFR is a measurement of the pressure drop over a stenosis. The larger the drop, the more functionally significant the stenosis is. It has been demonstrated that this value can be simulated using two orthogonal projection images and computational fluid dynamics [Morr 13, Tu 14, Trob 16]. This could be extended to make use of the better geometric accuracy and full coronary tree coverage of the 3-D reconstruction provided by RMC. First ideas for such an approach were laid out in [Laur 15]. Using the results from [Itu 16] that make use of machine learning instead of flow simulation, the determination of the FFR values could even be performed in real time.

Beyond geometrical information, there is also potential for clinical insight from the motion model itself. Motion defects of the heart are an indication for damage of the muscle, e.g. from a heart attack [Mull 14a]. Since the coronary arteries surround the heart muscle, their movement might be a sufficient approximation for similar studies. Several approaches how to animate a single-phase reconstruction have already been published [Hans 09, Holu 11], they would need to be extended for the 2-D motion model used in this work.

Finally, going beyond coronary artery reconstruction, post-implantation device evaluation is an interesting topic [Rodr 14, Rodr 15]. In these two publications, NOP-MEC was successfully employed. As demonstrated by Figure 1.3, device reconstruction is already feasible with RMC out of the box with a quality at least equivalent to NOPMEC, but surely deserves a separate, more careful investigation.

List of Symbols

List of Figures

List of Tables

List of Algorithms

Bibliography

[Ache 00] S. Achenbach, D. Ropers, J. Holle, G. Muschiol, W. Daniel, and W. Moshage. "In-Plane Coronary Arterial Motion Velocity: Measurement with Electron-Beam CT". *Radiology*, Vol. 216, No. 2, pp. 457–463, August 2000.

[Ache 12] S. Achenbach, V. Delgado, J. Hausleiter, P. Schoenhagen, J. K. Min, and J. A. Leipsic. "SCCT expert consensus document on computed tomography imaging before transcatheter aortic valve implantation (TAVI)/transcatheter aortic valve replacement (TAVR)". *J. Cardiovasc. Comput. Tomogr.*, Vol. 6, No. 6, pp. 366–380, November 2012.

[Addy 15] N. Addy, R. Reeve Ingle, H. Wu, B. Hu, and D. Nishimura. "High-resolution variable-density 3D cones coronary MRA". *Magn. Reson. Med.*, Vol. 74, No. 3, pp. 614–621, July 2015.

[Aren 15] R. Arena, M. Guazzi, L. Lianov, L. Whitsel, K. Berra, C. J. Lavie, L. Kaminsky, M. Williams, M.-F. Hivert, N. Cherie Franklin, *et al.* "Healthy lifestyle interventions to combat noncommunicable disease – a novel nonhierarchical connectivity model for key stakeholders: a policy statement from the American Heart Association, European Society of Cardiology, European Association for Cardiovascular Prevention and Rehabilitation, and American College of Preventive Medicine". *Eur. Heart J.*, Vol. 36, No. 31, pp. 2097–2109, July 2015.

[Aust 75] W. Austen, J. Edwards, R. Frye, G. Gensini, V. Gott, L. Griffith, D. McGoon, M. Murphy, and B. Roe. "A reporting system on patients evaluated for coronary artery disease". *Circulation*, Vol. 51, No. 4, pp. 5–40, April 1975.

[Beck 08] A. Becker, A. Leber, C. Becker, and A. Knez. "Predictive value of coronary calcifications for future cardiac events in asymptomatic individuals". *Am. Heart J.*, Vol. 155, No. 1, pp. 154–160, January 2008.

[Berg 14] M. Berger, C. Forman, C. Schwemmer, J.-H. Choi, K. Müller, A. Maier, J. Hornegger, and R. Fahrig. "Automatic Removal of Externally Attached Fiducial Markers in Cone Beam C-arm CT". In: H. H. and T. Deserno, Eds., *Bildverarbeitung für die Medizin 2014*, pp. 168–173, Aachen, Germany, March 2014.

[Blon 04] C. Blondel, G. Malandain, V. Régis, and A. Nicholas. "Reconstruction of coronary arteries from one rotational x-ray projection sequence". Research Report 5214, Sophia Antipolis: INRIA, May 2004.

[Blon 06] C. Blondel, G. Malandain, R. Vaillant, and N. Ayache. "Reconstruction of coronary arteries from a single rotational X-ray projection sequence". *IEEE Trans. Med. Imaging*, Vol. 25, No. 5, pp. 653–663, May 2006.

[Buzu 08] T. Buzug. *Computed Tomography – From Photon Statistics to Modern Cone-Beam CT*. Springer Verlag Berlin Heidelberg, 1st Ed., June 2008.

[Camm 10] J. Cammin and K. Taguchi. "Motion compensated filtered backprojection for non-rigid deformation". In: F. Noo, Ed., *Proc. 1st intl. conf. on image formation in X-ray CT*, pp. 162–165, Salt Lake City, UT, USA, June 2010.

[Camp 14] P. Campbell and E. Mahmud. "TCT-84 Prospective, Online, Interactive Survey Comparing Visual Lesion Estimation To Quantitative Coronary Angiography". In: *Proc. TCT 2014*, p. B25, CRF, Am. Coll. Cardio. Found., Washington D.C., USA, September 2014.

[Carr 09] J. Carroll, E. Carroll, and S. Chen. "Coronary Angiography: The Need for Improvement and the Barriers to Adoption of New Technology". *Cardiol. Clin.*, Vol. 27, No. 3, pp. 373–383, August 2009.

[Ceti 16] M. Cetin and A. Iskurt. "An Automatic 3-D Reconstruction of Coronary Arteries by Stereopsis". *J. Med. Syst.*, Vol. 40, No. 4, pp. 1–11, February 2016.

[Cham 83] J. Chambers, W. Cleveland, B. Kleiner, and P. Tukey. *Graphical Methods for Data Analysis. Chapman and Hall Statistics Series*, Wadsworth International Group, 1st Ed., February 1983.

[Chen 00] S.-Y. Chen and J. Carroll. "3-D reconstruction of coronary arterial tree to optimize angiographic visualization". *IEEE Trans. Med. Imaging*, Vol. 19, No. 4, pp. 318–336, April 2000.

[Chen 02] S.-Y. Chen, J. Carroll, and J. Messenger. "Quantitative analysis of reconstructed 3-D coronary arterial tree and intracoronary devices". *IEEE Trans. Med. Imaging*, Vol. 21, No. 7, pp. 724–740, July 2002.

[Chen 03] S.-Y. Chen and J. Carroll. "Kinematic and deformation analysis of 4-D coronary arterial trees reconstructed from cine angiograms". *IEEE Trans. Med. Imaging*, Vol. 22, No. 6, pp. 710–721, June 2003.

[Chen 09] S.-Y. Chen and D. Schäfer. "Three-dimensional coronary visualization, Part 1: modeling". *Cardiol. Clin.*, Vol. 27, No. 3, pp. 433–452, August 2009.

[Cime 16] S. Çimen, A. Gooya, M. Grass, and A. Frangi. "Reconstruction of Coronary Arteries from X-ray Angiography: A Review". *Med. Image Anal.*, Vol. 32, pp. 46–68, August 2016.

[Cong 15] W. Cong, J. Yang, D. Ai, Y. Chen, Y. Liu, and Y. Wang. "Quantitative Analysis of Deformable Model-Based 3-D Reconstruction of Coronary Artery From Multiple Angiograms". *IEEE Trans. Biomed. Eng.*, Vol. 62, No. 8, pp. 2079–2090, August 2015.

[Conr 03] R. Conroy, K. Pyörälä, A. Fitzgerald, S. Sans, A. Menotti, G. De Backer, D. De Bacquer, P. Ducimetiere, P. Jousilahti, U. Keil, *et al.* "Estimation of ten-year risk of fatal cardiovascular disease in Europe: the SCORE project". *Eur. Heart J.*, Vol. 24, No. 11, pp. 987–1003, June 2003.

[Desj 04] B. Desjardins and E. Kazerooni. "ECG-gated cardiac CT". *Am. J. Roentgenol.*, Vol. 182, No. 4, pp. 993–1010, April 2004.

[Ding 15] M. Ding, A. Satija, S. Bhupathiraju, Y. Hu, Q. Sun, J. Han, E. Lopez-Garcia, W. Willett, R. van Dam, and F. Hu. "Association of Coffee Consumption with Total and Cause-Specific Mortality in Three Large Prospective Cohorts". *Circulation*, Vol. 132, No. 24, pp. 2305–2315, December 2015.

[Dodg 92]   J. Dodge, B. Brown, E. Bolson, and H. Dodge. "Lumen diameter of normal human coronary arteries. Influence of age, sex, anatomic variation, and left ventricular hypertrophy or dilation.". *Circulation*, Vol. 86, No. 1, pp. 232–246, July 1992.

[Dori 13]   M. Döring, F. Braunschweig, C. Eitel, T. Gaspar, U. Wetzel, B. Nitsche, G. Hindricks, and C. Piorkowski. "Individually tailored left ventricular lead placement: lessons from multimodality integration between three-dimensional echocardiography and coronary sinus angiogram". *Europace*, Vol. 15, No. 5, pp. 718–727, February 2013.

[Doug 03]   E. Dougherty and R. Lotufo. *Hands-on Morphological Image Processing*. Vol. TT59 of *Tutorial Texts in Optical Engineering*, SPIE, Bellingham, WA, USA, July 2003.

[Egge 16]   H. Eggebrecht and R. Mehta. "Transcatheter aortic valve implantation (TAVI) in Germany 2008–2014: on its way to standard therapy for aortic valve stenosis in the elderly?". *EuroIntervention*, Vol. 11, No. 9, pp. 1029–1033, January 2016.

[Eng 13]   M. Eng, P. Hudson, A. Klein, S. Chen, M. Kim, B. Groves, J. Messenger, O. Wink, J. Carroll, and J. Garcia. "Impact of three dimensional in-room imaging (3DCA) in the facilitation of percutaneous coronary interventions". *J. Cardio. Vasc. Med.*, Vol. 1, No. 101, pp. 1–5, August 2013.

[Fahr 97]   R. Fahrig, A. J. Fox, S. Lownie, and D. W. Holdsworth. "Use of a C-arm system to generate true three-dimensional computed rotational angiograms: preliminary in vitro and in vivo results". *Am. J. Neurorad.*, Vol. 18, No. 8, pp. 1507–1514, September 1997.

[Fall 08]   P. Fallavollita and F. Cheriet. "Optimal 3D reconstruction of coronary arteries for 3D clinical assessment". *Comput. Med. Imaging Graph.*, Vol. 32, No. 6, pp. 476–487, September 2008.

[Feld 84]   L. Feldkamp, L. Davis, and J. Kress. "Practical cone-beam algorithm". *J. Opt. Soc. Am. A*, Vol. 1, No. 6, pp. 612–619, June 1984.

[Fitz 96]   A. W. Fitzgibbon, M. Pilu, and R. B. Fischer. "Direct least squares fitting of ellipses". In: *Proc. of the 13th International Conference on Pattern Recognition*, pp. 253–257, Vienna, Austria, September 1996.

[Form 13]   C. Forman, R. Grimm, J. Hutter, A. Maier, J. Hornegger, and M. Zenge. "Free-Breathing Whole-Heart Coronary MRA: Motion Compensation Integrated into 3D Cartesian Compressed Sensing Reconstruction". In: K. Mori, I. Sakuma, Y. Sato, C. Barillot, and N. Navab, Eds., *Medical Image Computing and Computer-Assisted Intervention – MICCAI 2013*, pp. 575–582, Springer, Nagoya, JP, September 2013.

[Form 14]   C. Forman, D. Piccini, R. Grimm, J. Hutter, J. Hornegger, and M. Zenge. "High-Resolution 3D Whole-Heart Coronary MRA: A Study on the Combination of Data Acquisition in Multiple Breath-Holds and 1D Residual Respiratory Motion Compensation". *Magn. Reson. Mater. Phy.*, Vol. 27, No. 5, pp. 435–443, October 2014.

[Fran 98]   A. Frangi, W. Niessen, K. Vincken, and M. Viergever. "Multiscale vessel enhancement filtering". In: W. Wells, A. Colchester, and S. Delp, Eds., *Medical Image Computing and Computer-Assisted Intervention –*

          MICCAI 1998, pp. 130–137, Springer, Cambridge, MA, USA, October
          1998.

[Frim 08] O. Friman, M. Hindennach, and H.-O. Peitgen. "Template-based Multiple
          Hypotheses Tracking of Small Vessels". In: *5th International Symposium
          on Biomedical Imaging: From Nano to Macro (ISBI 2008)*, pp. 1047–
          1050, IEEE, Paris, France, May 2008.

[Gali 03] R. Galigekere, K. Wiesent, and D. Holdsworth. "Cone-beam Reprojection
          Using Projection-Matrices". *IEEE Trans. Med. Imaging*, Vol. 22, No. 10,
          pp. 1202–1214, September 2003.

[Garc 09] J. Garcia, S. Bhakta, J. Kay, K.-C. Chan, O. Wink, D. Ruijters, and
          J. Carroll. "On-line multi-slice computed tomography interactive overlay
          with conventional X-ray: a new and advanced imaging fusion concept".
          Int. J. Cardiol., Vol. 133, No. 3, pp. e101–e105, April 2009.

[Goll 07] R. Gollapudi, R. Valencia, S. Lee, G. Wong, P. Teirstein, and M. Price.
          "Utility of three-dimensional reconstruction of coronary angiography to
          guide percutaneous coronary intervention". *Catheter. Cardiovasc. Interv.*,
          Vol. 69, No. 4, pp. 479–482, March 2007.

[Gray 00] H. Gray. *Anatomy of the Human Body*. Lea & Febiger, Philadelphia,
          USA (1918). Bartleby.com, New York, USA, 20th Ed., May 2000.

[Gree 04] N. Green, S.-Y. Chen, J. Messenger, B. Groves, and J. Carroll. "Three-
          dimensional vascular angiography". *Curr. Probl. Cardiol.*, Vol. 29, No. 3,
          pp. 104–142, March 2004.

[Gutl 11] K.-J. Gutleben, G. Nölker, G. Ritscher, H. Rittger, C. Rohkohl, G. Laur-
          itsch, J. Brachmann, and A. M. Sina. "Three-dimensional coronary si-
          nus reconstruction-guided left ventricular lead implantation based on in-
          traprocedural rotational angiography: a novel imaging modality in car-
          diac resynchronisation device implantation". *Europace*, Vol. 13, No. 5,
          pp. 675–682, February 2011.

[Hali 98] R. Halir and J. Flusser. "Numerically stable direct least squares fit-
          ting of ellipses". In: N. Thalmann and V. Skala, Eds., *6th International
          Conference in Central Europe on Computer Graphics and Visualization
          (WSCG)*, pp. 125–132, Plzen - Bory, Czech Republic, February 1998.

[Hamm 11] C. W. Hamm, J.-P. Bassand, S. Agewall, J. Bax, E. Boersma, H. Bueno,
          P. Caso, D. Dudek, S. Gielen, K. Huber, *et al.* "ESC Guidelines for the
          management of acute coronary syndromes in patients presenting without
          persistent ST-segment elevation". *Eur. Heart J.*, Vol. 32, No. 23, pp. 2999–
          3054, August 2011.

[Hans 08a] E. Hansis, D. Schäfer, O. Dössel, and M. Grass. "Evaluation of iterat-
          ive sparse object reconstruction from few projections for 3-D rotational
          coronary angiography". *IEEE Trans. Med. Imaging*, Vol. 27, No. 11,
          pp. 1548–1555, November 2008.

[Hans 08b] E. Hansis, D. Schäfer, O. Dössel, and M. Grass. "Projection-based motion
          compensation for gated coronary artery reconstruction from rotational x-
          ray angiograms". *Phys. Med. Biol.*, Vol. 53, No. 14, pp. 3807–3820, June
          2008.

[Hans 09]   E. Hansis, H. Schomberg, K. Erhard, O. Dössel, and M. Grass. "Four-Dimensional Cardiac Reconstruction from Rotational X-ray Sequences: First Results for 4D Coronary Angiography". In: E. Samei and J. Hsieh, Eds., *SPIE Medical Imaging: Physics of Medical Imaging*, pp. 72580B–72580B–11, SPIE, Lake Buena Vista, FL, USA, February 2009.

[Hech 15]   H. S. Hecht. "Coronary Artery Calcium Scanning". *JACC: Cardiovasc. Imag.*, Vol. 8, No. 5, pp. 579–596, May 2015.

[Hell 14]   M. M. Hell, D. Bittner, A. Schuhbaeck, G. Muschiol, M. Brand, M. Lell, M. Uder, S. Achenbach, and M. Marwan. "Prospectively ECG-triggered high-pitch coronary angiography with third-generation dual-source CT at 70 kVp tube voltage: Feasibility, image quality, radiation dose, and effect of iterative reconstruction". *J. Cardiovasc. Comput. Tomogr.*, Vol. 8, No. 6, pp. 418–425, November 2014.

[Hett 10]   H. Hetterich, T. Redel, G. Lauritsch, C. Rohkohl, and J. Rieber. "New X-ray imaging modalities and their integration with intravascular imaging and interventions". *Int. J. Cardiovas. Imag.*, Vol. 26, No. 7, pp. 797–808, October 2010.

[Hofm 11]   H. G. Hofmann, B. Keck, C. Rohkohl, and J. Hornegger. "Comparing performance of many-core CPUs and GPUs for static and motion compensated reconstruction of C-arm CT data". *Med. Phys.*, Vol. 38, No. 1, pp. 468–473, January 2011.

[Hohl 08]   C. Hohl, J. Boese, N. Strobel, R. Banckwitz, G. Lauritsch, G. Mühlenbruch, and R. Günther. "Angiographische CT: Messung der Patientendosis". In: D. Vorwerk and R. Fotter, Eds., *89. Deutscher Röntgenkongress*, DRG, ÖRG, Thieme Publishing Group, Berlin, Germany, April/May 2008.

[Holu 11]   W. Holub, C. Rohkohl, D. Schuldhaus, M. Prümmer, G. Lauritsch, and J. Hornegger. "4D motion animation of coronary arteries from rotational angiography". In: K. Wong and D. I. Holmes, Eds., *SPIE Medical Imaging: Visualization, Image-Guided Procedures, and Modeling*, pp. 79641S–79641S–10, SPIE, Lake Buena Vista, Florida, USA, February 2011.

[Husm 07]   L. Husmann, S. Leschka, L. Desbiolles, T. Schepis, O. Gaemperli, B. Seifert, P. Cattin, T. Frauenfelder, T. Flohr, B. Marincek, P. Kaufmann, and H. Alkadhi. "Coronary Artery Motion and Cardiac Phases: Dependency on Heart Rate – Implications for CT Image Reconstruction". *Radiology*, Vol. 245, No. 2, pp. 567–576, November 2007.

[Isol 10]   A. A. Isola, M. Grass, and W. J. Niessen. "Fully automatic nonrigid registration-based local motion estimation for motion-corrected iterative cardiac CT reconstruction". *Med. Phys.*, Vol. 37, No. 3, pp. 1093–1109, March 2010.

[Itu 16]   L. Itu, S. Rapaka, T. Passerini, B. Georgescu, C. Schwemmer, M. Schoebinger, T. Flohr, P. Sharma, and D. Comaniciu. "A machine-learning approach for computation of fractional flow reserve from coronary computed tomography". *J. Appl. Physiol.*, Vol. 121, No. 1, pp. 42–52, July 2016.

[Jand 09a]   U. Jandt, D. Schäfer, M. Grass, and V. Rasche. "Automatic generation of 3D coronary artery centerlines using rotational X-ray angiography". *Med. Image Anal.*, Vol. 13, No. 6, pp. 846–858, December 2009.

[Jand 09b] U. Jandt, D. Schäfer, M. Grass, and V. Rasche. "Automatic generation of time resolved motion vector fields of coronary arteries and 4D surface extraction using rotational x-ray angiography". *Phys. Med. Biol.*, Vol. 54, No. 1, pp. 45–64, January 2009.

[Keil 09] A. Keil, J. Vogel, G. Lauritsch, and N. Navab. "Dynamic Cone Beam Reconstruction Using a New Level Set Formulation". In: G.-Z. Yang, D. Hawkes, D. Rueckert, A. Noble, and C. Taylor, Eds., *Medical Image Computing and Computer-Assisted Intervention – MICCAI 2009*, pp. 389–397, Springer, London, UK, September 2009.

[Kern 06] M. Kern, A. Lerman, J.-W. Bech, B. De Bruyne, E. Eeckhout, W. Fearon, S. Higano, M. Lim, M. Meuwissen, J. Piek, *et al.* "Physiological Assessment of Coronary Artery Disease in the Cardiac Catheterization Laboratory: A Scientific Statement From the American Heart Association Committee on Diagnostic and Interventional Cardiac Catheterization, Council on Clinical Cardiology". *Circulation*, Vol. 114, No. 12, pp. 1321–1341, September 2006.

[Krak 04] I. Krakau and H. Lapp. *Das Herzkatheterbuch: diagnostische und interventionelle Kathetertechniken.* Thieme, Stuttgart, DE, 2nd Ed., November 2004. p. 38.

[Laur 15] G. Lauritsch, T. Redel, M. Scheuering, and C. Schwemmer. "FLUID-DYNAMIC ANALYSIS OF A VASCULAR TREE USING ANGIOGRAPHY". Patent US2015356753 (A1), December 2015.

[Lebo 11] A. Lebois, R. Florent, and V. Auvray. "Geometry-constrained coronary arteries motion estimation from 2D angiograms – Application to injection side recognition". In: S. Wright, X. Pan, and M. Liebling, Eds., *8th International Symposium on Biomedical Imaging: From Nano to Macro (ISBI 2011)*, pp. 541–544, IEEE, Chicago, IL, USA, March 2011.

[Lehm 06] G. Lehmann, D. Holdsworth, and M. Drangova. "Angle-independent measure of motion for image-based gating in 3D coronary angiography". *Med. Phys.*, Vol. 33, No. 5, pp. 1311–1320, April 2006.

[Li 01] D. Li, J. Carr, S. Shea, J. Zheng, V. Deshpande, P. Wielopolski, and J. Finn. "Coronary Arteries: Magnetization-prepared Contrast-enhanced Threedimensional Volume-targeted Breath-hold MR Angiography". *Radiology*, Vol. 219, No. 1, pp. 270–277, April 2001.

[Like 32] R. Likert. "A technique for the measurement of attitudes". *Archives of psychology*, Vol. 22, No. 140, p. 55, 1932.

[Lore 04] C. Lorenz, J. von Berg, T. Bülow, S. Renisch, and S. Wergandt. "Modeling the coronary artery tree". In: *Proc. Shape Modeling Applications*, IEEE, Genova, Italy, June 2004.

[Lu 01] B. Lu, S.-S. Mao, N. Zhuang, H. Bakhsheshi, H. Yamamoto, J. Takasu, S. C. Liu, and M. J. Budoff. "Coronary artery motion during the cardiac cycle and optimal ECG triggering for coronary artery imaging". *Invest. Radiol.*, Vol. 36, No. 5, pp. 250–256, May 2001.

[Ma 12] Y. Ma, A. Shetty, S. Duckett, P. Etyngier, G. Gijsbers, R. Bullens, T. Schaeffter, R. Razavi, C. Rinaldi, and K. Rhode. "An integrated platform for image-guided cardiac resynchronization therapy". *Phys. Med. Biol.*, Vol. 57, No. 10, pp. 2953–2968, April 2012.

[Madd 04]   J. T. Maddux, O. Wink, J. C. Messenger, B. M. Groves, R. Liao, J. Strzel-czyk, S.-Y. Chen, and J. D. Carroll. "Randomized study of the safety and clinical utility of rotational angiography versus standard angiography in the diagnosis of coronary artery disease". *Catheter. Cardiovasc. Interv.*, Vol. 62, No. 2, pp. 167–174, May 2004.

[Maie 12]   A. Maier, H. G. Hofmann, C. Schwemmer, J. Hornegger, A. Keil, and R. Fahrig. "Fast simulation of x-ray projections of spline-based surfaces using an append buffer". *Phys. Med. Biol.*, Vol. 57, No. 19, pp. 6193–6210, September 2012.

[Maie 13]   A. Maier, H. G. Hofmann, M. Berger, P. Fischer, C. Schwemmer, H. Wu, K. Müller, J. Hornegger, J.-W. Choi, C. Riess, A. Keil, and R. Fahrig. "CONRAD – A software framework for cone-beam imaging in radiology". *Med. Phys.*, Vol. 40, No. 11, p. 111914, October 2013.

[Mark 10]   D. Mark, D. Berman, M. Budoff, J. Carr, T. Gerber, H. Hecht, M. Hlatky, J. Hodgson, M. Lauer, J. Miller, *et al.* "ACCF/ACR/AHA/NASCI/SAIP/SCAI/SCCT 2010 Expert Consensus Document on Coronary Computed Tomographic Angiography". *J. Am. Coll. Cardiol.*, Vol. 55, No. 23, pp. 2663–2699, June 2010.

[McCu 08]   P. McCullough. "Contrast-Induced Acute Kidney Injury". *J. Am. Coll. Cardiol.*, Vol. 51, No. 15, pp. 1419–1428, April 2008.

[Mont 13]   G. Montalescot, U. Sechtem, S. Achenbach, F. Andreotti, C. Arden, A. Budaj, R. Bugiardini, F. Crea, T. Cuisset, C. Di Mario, *et al.* "2013 ESC guidelines on the management of stable coronary artery disease". *Eur Heart J*, Vol. 34, No. 38, pp. 2949–3003, August 2013.

[Morr 13]   P. Morris, D. Ryan, A. Morton, R. Lycett, P. Lawford, D. Hose, and J. Gunn. "Virtual Fractional Flow Reserve From Coronary Angiography: Modeling the Significance of Coronary Lesions: Results From the VIRTU-1 (VIRTUal Fractional Flow Reserve From Coronary Angiography) Study". *JACC: Cardiovascular Interventions*, Vol. 6, No. 2, pp. 149–157, February 2013.

[Morr 15]   P. Morris, J. Taylor, S. Boutong, S. Brett, A. Louis, J. Heppenstall, A. Morton, and J. Gunn. "When is rotational angiography superior to conventional single-plane angiography for planning coronary angioplasty?". *Cathet. Cardiovasc. Intervent.*, Vol. 87, No. 4, pp. E104–E112, May 2015.

[Mors 14]   F. Morsbach, S. Gordic, L. Desbiolles, D. Husarik, T. Frauenfelder, B. Schmidt, T. Allmendinger, S. Wildermuth, H. Alkadhi, and S. Leschka. "Performance of turbo high-pitch dual-source CT for coronary CT angiography: first ex vivo and patient experience". *Eur. Radiol.*, Vol. 24, No. 8, pp. 1889–1895, May 2014.

[Mova 03]   B. Movassaghi, V. Rasche, R. Florent, M. Viergever, and W. Niessen. "3D coronary reconstruction from calibrated motion-compensated 2D projections". In: *Proc. of CARS*, pp. 1079–1084, Elsevier BV, London, UK, June 2003.

[Mova 04]   B. Movassaghi, V. Rasche, M. Grass, M. Viergever, and W. Niessen. "A quantitative analysis of 3-D coronary modeling from two or more projection images". *IEEE Trans. Med. Imaging*, Vol. 23, No. 12, pp. 1517–1531, December 2004.

[Moza 15]   D. Mozaffarian, E. Benjamin, A. Go, D. Arnett, M. Blaha, M. Cushman, S. de Ferranti, J.-P. Després, H. Fullerton, V. Howard, *et al.* "Heart Disease and Stroke Statistics–2015 Update: A Report From the American Heart Association". *Circulation*, Vol. 131, No. 4, pp. e29–e322, January 2015.

[Mull 12]   K. Müller, C. Rohkohl, G. Lauritsch, C. Schwemmer, H. Heidbüchel, S. De Buck, D. Nuyens, Y. Kyriakou, C. Köhler, and J. Hornegger. "4-D Motion Field Estimation by Combined Multiple Heart Phase Registration (CMHPR) for Cardiac C-arm Data". In: *IEEE NSS/MIC Record*, pp. 3707–3712, Anaheim, CA, USA, November 2012.

[Mull 13]   K. Müller, C. Schwemmer, J. Hornegger, Y. Zheng, Y. Wang, G. Lauritsch, C. Rohkohl, A. Maier, C. Schultz, and R. Fahrig. "Evaluation of interpolation methods for surface-based motion compensated tomographic reconstruction for cardiac angiographic C-arm data". *Med. Phys.*, Vol. 40, No. 3, pp. 031107-1–12, February 2013.

[Mull 14a] K. Müller. *3-D Imaging of the Heart Chambers with C-arm CT*. PhD thesis, Technische Fakultät, Universität Erlangen-Nürnberg, May 2014.

[Mull 14b] K. Müller, G. Lauritsch, C. Schwemmer, A. Maier, O. Taubmann, B. Abt, H. Köhler, A. Nöttling, J. Hornegger, and R. Fahrig. "Catheter artifact reduction (CAR) in dynamic cardiac chamber imaging with interventional C-arm CT". In: F. Noo, Ed., *Proc. 3rd intl. mtg. on image formation in X-ray CT*, pp. 418–421, Salt Lake City, UT, USA, June 2014.

[Mull 14c] K. Müller, A. Maier, C. Schwemmer, G. Lauritsch, S. De Buck, J.-Y. Wielandts, J. Hornegger, and R. Fahrig. "Image artefact propagation in motion estimation and reconstruction in interventional cardiac C-arm CT". *Phys. Med. Biol.*, Vol. 59, No. 12, pp. 3121–3138, June 2014.

[Newb 15]   D. Newby, P. Mannucci, G. Tell, A. Baccarelli, R. Brook, K. Donaldson, F. Forastiere, M. Franchini, O. Franco, I. Graham, *et al.* "Expert position paper on air pollution and cardiovascular disease". *Eur. Heart J.*, Vol. 36, No. 2, pp. 83–93, December 2015.

[Niem 01]   K. Nieman, M. Oudkerk, B. Rensing, P. van Ooijen, A. Munne, R.-J. van Geuns, and P. de Feyter. "Coronary angiography with multi-slice computed tomography". *The Lancet*, Vol. 357, No. 9256, pp. 599–603, February 2001.

[Onum 11]   Y. Onuma, C. Girasis, J.-P. Aben, G. Sarno, N. Piazza, C. Lokkerbol, M.-A. Morel, and P. Serruys. "A novel dedicated 3-dimensional quantitative coronary analysis methodology for bifurcation lesions". *EuroIntervention*, Vol. 7, No. 5, pp. 629–635, September 2011.

[Orth 09]   R. Orth, M. Wallace, and M. Kuo. "C-arm Cone-beam CT: General Principles and Technical Considerations for Use in Interventional Radiology". *J. Vasc. Interv. Radiol.*, Vol. 19, No. 6, pp. 814–820, June 2009.

[Perk 12]   J. Perk, G. De Backer, H. Gohlke, I. Graham, Ž. Reiner, M. Verschuren, C. Albus, P. Benlian, G. Boysen, R. Cifkova, *et al.* "European Guidelines on cardiovascular disease prevention in clinical practice (version 2012)". *Eur. Heart J.*, Vol. 33, No. 13, pp. 1635–1701, May 2012.

[Perr 07]   B. Perrenot, R. Vaillant, R. Prost, G. Finet, P. Douek, and F. Peyrin. "Motion correction for coronary stent reconstruction from rotational X-ray projection sequences". *IEEE Trans. Med. Imaging*, Vol. 26, No. 10, pp. 1412–1423, October 2007.

[Picc 12]   D. Piccini, A. Littmann, S. Nielles-Vallespin, and M. Zenge. "Respiratory self-navigation for whole-heart bright-blood coronary MRI: Methods for robust isolation and automatic segmentation of the blood pool". *Magn. Reson. Med.*, Vol. 68, No. 2, pp. 571–579, August 2012.

[Pijl 07]   N. Pijls, P. van Schaardenburgh, G. Manoharan, E. Boersma, J.-W. Bech, M. van't Veer, F. Bär, J. Hoorntje, J. Koolen, W. Wijns, and B. de Bruyne. "Percutaneous Coronary Intervention of Functionally Nonsignificant Stenosis: 5-year follow-up of the DEFER Study". *J. Am. Coll. Cardiol.*, Vol. 49, No. 21, pp. 2105–2111, May 2007.

[Poly 12]   M. Polyanskaya, C. Schwemmer, A. G. Linarth, J. Hornegger, and G. Lauritsch. "Robust Lumen Segmentation of Coronary Arteries in 2D Angiographic Images". In: D. Haynor and S. Ourselin, Eds., *SPIE Medical Imaging: Image Processing*, pp. 83142N–1–7, SPIE, San Diego, CA, USA, February 2012.

[Prum 09]   M. Prümmer, J. Hornegger, G. Lauritsch, L. Wigström, E. Girard-Hughes, and R. Fahrig. "Cardiac C-Arm CT: A Unified Framework for Motion Estimation and Dynamic CT". *IEEE Trans. Med. Imaging*, Vol. 28, No. 11, pp. 1836–49, October 2009.

[Rasc 04]   V. Rasche, B. Movassaghi, and M. Grass. "Automatic gating window selection for gated three-dimensional coronary X-ray angiography". In: *Proc. of CARS*, pp. 1050–1054, Chicago, IL, USA, June 2004.

[Rasc 06]   V. Rasche, B. Movassaghi, M. Grass, D. Schäfer, and A. Buecker. "Automatic Selection of the Optimal Cardiac Phase for Gated Three-dimensional Coronary x-ray Angiography". *Acad. Radiol.*, Vol. 13, No. 5, pp. 630–640, May 2006.

[Rodr 14]   R. Rodríguez-Olivares, N. Van Mieghem, and P. De Jaegere. "The Role of Frame Geometry Assessment During Transcatheter Aortic Valve Replacement by Rotational Angiography". *JACC: Cardiovascular Interventions*, Vol. 7, No. 12, pp. e191–e192, December 2014.

[Rodr 15]   R. Rodríguez-Olivares, N. El Faquir, Z. Rahhab, P. Geeve, A. Maugenest, S. van Weenen, B. Ren, T. Galema, M. Geleijnse, N. Van Mieghem, *et al.* "Does frame geometry play a role in aortic regurgitation after Medtronic CoreValve implantation?". *EuroIntervention*, Vol. 11, No. 4, pp. 1–12, August 2015.

[Rohk 08a]   C. Rohkohl, M. Prümmer, R. Fahrig, G. Lauritsch, and J. Hornegger. "Cardiac C-arm CT: image-based gating". In: J. Hsieh and E. Samei, Eds., *SPIE Medical Imaging: Image Processing*, pp. 69131G–1–12, SPIE, San Diego, CA, USA, February 2008.

[Rohk 08b]   C. Rohkohl, G. Lauritsch, A. Nöttling, M. Prümmer, and J. Hornegger. "C-Arm CT: Reconstruction of Dynamic High Contrast Objects Applied to the Coronary Sinus". In: *IEEE NSS/MIC Record*, pp. M10–328, Dresden, Germany, October 2008.

[Rohk 09a] C. Rohkohl, B. Keck, H. Hofmann, and J. Hornegger. "Technical Note: RabbitCT – an open platform for benchmarking 3D cone-beam reconstruction algorithms". *Med. Phys.*, Vol. 36, No. 9, pp. 3940–3944, September 2009.

[Rohk 09b] C. Rohkohl, G. Lauritsch, M. Prümmer, and J. Hornegger. "Interventional 4-D motion estimation and reconstruction of cardiac vasculature without motion periodicity assumption". In: G.-Z. Yang, D. Hawkes, D. Rueckert, A. Noble, and C. Taylor, Eds., *Medical Image Computing and Computer-Assisted Intervention – MICCAI 2009*, pp. 132–9, Springer, London, UK, September 2009.

[Rohk 10a] C. Rohkohl, G. Lauritsch, L. Biller, and J. Hornegger. "ECG-gated Interventional Cardiac Reconstruction for Non-periodic Motion". In: T. Jiang, N. Navab, J. Pluim, and M. Viergever, Eds., *Medical Image Computing and Computer-Assisted Intervention – MICCAI 2010*, pp. 151–158, Springer, Beijing, China, September 2010.

[Rohk 10b] C. Rohkohl, G. Lauritsch, L. Biller, M. Prümmer, J. Boese, and J. Hornegger. "Interventional 4D motion estimation and reconstruction of cardiac vasculature without motion periodicity assumption". *Medical Image Analysis*, Vol. 14, No. 5, pp. 687–694, October 2010.

[Rohk 10c] C. Rohkohl, G. Lauritsch, A. Keil, and J. Hornegger. "CAVAREV – An Open Platform for Evaluating 3D and 4D Cardiac Vasculature Reconstruction". *Phys. Med. Biol.*, Vol. 55, No. 10, pp. 2905–2915, April 2010.

[Rohk 11] C. Rohkohl. *Motion Estimation and Compensation for Interventional Cardiovascular Image Reconstruction*. PhD thesis, Technische Fakultät, Universität Erlangen-Nürnberg, January 2011.

[Roug 93] A. Rougée, C. Picard, C. Ponchut, and Y. Trousset. "Geometrical calibration of x-ray imaging chains for three-dimensional reconstruction". *Comput. Med. Imaging Graph.*, Vol. 17, No. 4-5, pp. 295–300, October 1993.

[Ruij 08] D. Ruijters, B. ter Haar Romeny, and P. Suetens. "Efficient GPU-Based Texture Interpolation using Uniform B-Splines". *Journal of Graphics, GPU, & Game Tools*, Vol. 13, No. 4, pp. 61–69, January 2008.

[Russ 03] D. Russakoff, T. Rohlfing, A. Ho, D. Kim, R. Shahidi, J. Adler, and C. Maurer. "Evaluation of Intensity-Based 2D–3D Spine Image Registration Using Clinical Gold-Standard Data". In: J. Gee, J. Maintz, and M. Vannier, Eds., *Second International Workshop on Biomedical Image Registration (WBIR 2003)*, pp. 151–160, Springer, Philadelphia, PA, USA, June 2003.

[Ruzs 09] B. Ruzsics, M. Gebregziabher, H. Lee, R. Brothers, T. Allmendinger, S. Vogt, P. Costello, and U. Schoepf. "Coronary CT angiography: automatic cardiac-phase selection for image reconstruction". *Eur. Radiol.*, Vol. 19, No. 8, pp. 1906–1913, March 2009.

[Sain 94] D. Saint-Félix, Y. Trousset, C. Picard, C. Ponchut, R. Roméas, and A. Rougée. "In vivo evaluation of a new system for 3D computerized angiography". *Phys. Med. Biol.*, Vol. 39, No. 3, pp. 583–595, March 1994.

[Scha 07]   D. Schäfer, B. Movassaghi, M. Grass, G. Schoonenberg, R. Florent, O. Wink, A. Klein, J. Chen, J. Garcia, J. Messenger, and J. Carroll. "Three-dimensional reconstruction of coronary stents in vivo based on motion compensated X-ray angiography". In: K. Cleary and M. Miga, Eds., *SPIE Medical Imaging: Visualization and Image-Guided Procedures*, pp. 65091M–1–8, SPIE, San Diego, CA, USA, February 2007.

[Scho 07]   H. Schomberg. "Time-Resolved Cardiac Cone Beam CT". In: *Proc. 9th Intl. Mtg. on Fully Three-Dimensional Image Reconstruction in Radiology and Nuclear Medicine*, pp. 362–365, Lindau, Germany, July 2007.

[Scho 09]   G. Schoonenberg, A. Neubauer, and M. Grass. "Three-Dimensional Coronary Visualization, Part 2: 3D Reconstruction". *Cardiol. Clin.*, Vol. 27, No. 3, pp. 453–465, August 2009.

[Schr 08]   S. Schroeder, S. Achenbach, F. Bengel, C. Burgstahler, F. Cademartiri, P. de Feyter, R. George, P. Kaufmann, A. F. Kopp, J. Knuuti, D. Ropers, J. Schuijf, L. F. Tops, and J. J. Bax. "Cardiac computed tomography: indications, applications, limitations, and training requirements". *Eur. Heart J.*, Vol. 29, No. 4, pp. 531–556, February 2008.

[Schw 10]   C. Schwemmer, M. Prümmer, V. Daum, and J. Hornegger. "High-Density Object Removal from Projection Images using Low-Frequency-Based Object Masking". In: T. Deserno, H. H., H.-P. Meinzer, and T. Tolxdorff, Eds., *Bildverarbeitung für die Medizin 2010 - Algorithmen - Systeme - Anwendungen*, pp. 365–369, Aachen, Germany, March 2010.

[Schw 12]   C. Schwemmer, C. Rohkohl, G. Lauritsch, K. Müller, and J. Hornegger. "Residual Motion Compensation in ECG-Gated Cardiac Vasculature Reconstruction". In: F. Noo, Ed., *Proc. 2nd intl. mtg. on image formation in X-ray CT*, pp. 259–262, Salt Lake City, UT, USA, June 2012.

[Schw 13a]   C. Schwemmer, C. Rohkohl, G. Lauritsch, K. Müller, and J. Hornegger. "Opening Windows – Increasing Window Size in Motion-Compensated ECG-gated Cardiac Vasculature Reconstruction". In: R. Leahy and J. Qi, Eds., *Proc. 12th Intl. Mtg. on Fully Three-Dimensional Image Reconstruction in Radiology and Nuclear Medicine*, pp. 50–53, Lake Tahoe, CA, USA, June 2013.

[Schw 13b]   C. Schwemmer, C. Rohkohl, G. Lauritsch, K. Müller, and J. Hornegger. "Residual Motion Compensation in ECG-Gated Interventional Cardiac Vasculature Reconstruction". *Phys. Med. Biol.*, Vol. 58, No. 11, pp. 3717–3737, May 2013.

[Schw 14a]   C. Schwemmer, C. Forman, J. Wetzl, A. Maier, and J. Hornegger. "Coro-Eval – A Multi-platform, Multi-modality Tool for the Evaluation of 3-D Coronary Vessel Reconstructions". *Phys. Med. Biol.*, Vol. 59, No. 17, pp. 5163–5174, September 2014.

[Schw 14b]   C. Schwemmer, G. Lauritsch, A. Kleinfeld, C. Rohkohl, K. Müller, and J. Hornegger. "Clinical Data Evaluation of C-arm-based Motion Compensated Coronary Artery Reconstruction". In: F. Noo, Ed., *Proc. 3rd intl. mtg. on image formation in X-ray CT*, pp. 60–63, Salt Lake City, UT, USA, June 2014.

[Schä 06]   D. Schäfer, J. Borgert, V. Rasche, and M. Grass. "Motion-compensated and gated cone beam filtered back-projection for 3-D rotational X-ray angiography". *IEEE Trans. Med. Imaging*, Vol. 25, No. 7, pp. 898–906, July 2006.

[Sega 01]   W.-P. Segars, D. Lalush, and B.-M.-W. Tsui. "Modelling Respiratory Mechanics in the MCAT and Spline-Based MCAT Phantoms". *IEEE Trans. Nucl. Sci.*, Vol. 48, No. 1, pp. 89–97, February 2001.

[Sega 08]   W.-P. Segars, M. Mahesh, T. Beck, E. Frey, and B.-M.-W. Tsui. "Realistic CT simulation using the 4D XCAT phantom". *Med. Phys.*, Vol. 35, No. 8, pp. 3800–3808, August 2008.

[Sega 99]   W.-P. Segars, D. Lalush, and B.-M.-W. Tsui. "A realistic spline-based dynamic heart phantom". *IEEE Trans. Nucl. Sci.*, Vol. 46, No. 3, pp. 503–506, June 1999.

[Serr 13]   P. Serruys. "TAVI in Europe – that was then and this is now". *EuroIntervention*, Vol. 9, No. 4, pp. 415–417, August 2013.

[Shaf 95]   J. Shaffer. "Multiple hypothesis testing". *Annu. Rev. Psychol.*, Vol. 46, No. 1, pp. 561–584, February 1995.

[Shap 00]   L. Shapiro and G. Stockman. *Computer Vision*. Prentice Hall, Upper Saddle River, NJ, USA, 1st Ed., March 2000.

[Stro 09]   N. Strobel, O. Meissner, J. Boese, T. Brunner, B. Heigl, M. Hoheisel, G. Lauritsch, M. Nagel, M. Pfister, E. P. Rührnschopf, *et al. Imaging with Flat-Detector C-Arm Systems*, Chap. 3, pp. 33–51. Springer Verlag Berlin Heidelberg, 3rd Ed., 2009.

[Suzu 13]   S. Suzuki, H. Machida, I. Tanaka, and E. Ueno. "Vascular Diameter Measurement in CT Angiography: Comparison of Model-Based Iterative Reconstruction and Standard Filtered Back Projection Algorithms In Vitro". *Am. J. Roentgenol.*, Vol. 200, No. 3, pp. 652–657, March 2013.

[Tagu 07]   K. Taguchi, Z. Sun, W.-P. Segars, E.-K. Fishman, and B.-M.-W. Tsui. "Image-domain motion compensated time resolved 4D cardiac CT". In: J. Hsieh and M. Flynn, Eds., *SPIE Medical Imaging: Physics of Medical Imaging*, pp. 651016–651016–9, SPIE, San Diego, CA, USA, February 2007.

[Tang 12]   Q. Tang, J. Cammin, S. Srivastava, and K. Taguchi. "A fully four-dimensional, iterative motion estimation and compensation method for cardiac CT". *Med. Phys.*, Vol. 39, No. 7, pp. 4291–4305, July 2012.

[Taub 15]   O. Taubmann, J. Wetzl, G. Lauritsch, A. Maier, and J. Hornegger. "Sharp as a Tack: Measuring and Comparing Edge Sharpness in Motion-Compensated Medical Image Reconstruction". In: H. Handels, T. Deserno, H.-P. Meinzer, and T. Tolxdorff, Eds., *Bildverarbeitung für die Medizin 2015 - Algorithmen - Systeme - Anwendungen*, pp. 425–430, Lübeck, DE, February 2015.

[Taub 16a] O. Taubmann, G. Lauritsch, G. Krings, and A. Maier. "Convex Temporal Regularizers in Cardiac C-arm CT". In: M. Kachelrieß, Ed., *Proc. 4th intl. mtg. on image formation in X-ray CT*, pp. 545–548, Bamberg, Germany, July 2016.

[Taub 16b] O. Taubmann, A. Maier, J. Hornegger, G. Lauritsch, and R. Fahrig. "Coping with Real World Data: Artifact Reduction and Denoising for Motion-Compensated Cardiac C-arm CT". *Med. Phys.*, Vol. 43, No. 2, pp. 883–893, January 2016.

[Taub 17] O. Taubmann, M. Unberath, G. Lauritsch, S. Achenbach, and A. Maier. "Spatio-temporally Regularized 4-D Cardiovascular C-arm CT Reconstruction Using a Proximal Algorithm". In: G. Egan and O. Salvado, Eds., *Proc. 2017 IEEE Intl. Symposium on Biomed. Imag. (ISBI)*, pp. 52–55, IEEE, Melbourne, Australia, April 2017.

[Tomm 98] G. Tommasini, A. Camerini, A. Gatti, G. Derchi, A. Bruzzone, and C. Vecchio. "Panoramic Coronary Angiography". *J. Am. Coll. Cardiol.*, Vol. 31, No. 4, pp. 871–877, March 1998.

[Trob 16] M. Tröbs, S. Achenbach, J. Röther, T. Redel, M. Scheuering, D. Winneberger, K. Klingenbeck, L. Itu, T. Passerini, A. Kamen, *et al.* "Comparison of Fractional Flow Reserve Based on Computational Fluid Dynamics Modeling Using Coronary Angiographic Vessel Morphology Versus Invasively Measured Fractional Flow Reserve". *The American Journal of Cardiology*, Vol. 117, No. 1, pp. 29–35, January 2016.

[Tu 14] S. Tu, E. Barbato, Z. Köszegi, J. Yang, Z. Sun, N. Holm, B. Tar, Y. Li, D. Rusinaru, W. Wijns, and J. Reiber. "Fractional Flow Reserve Calculation From 3-Dimensional Quantitative Coronary Angiography and TIMI Frame Count". *JACC: Cardiovasc. Intervent.*, Vol. 7, No. 7, pp. 768–777, July 2014.

[Turg 05] G.-A. Turgeon, G. Lehmann, G. Guiraudon, M. Drangova, D. Holdsworth, and T. Peters. "2D-3D registration of coronary angiograms for cardiac procedure planning and guidance". *Med. Phys.*, Vol. 32, No. 12, pp. 3737–3749, November 2005.

[Unbe 15] M. Unberath, K. Mentl, O. Taubmann, S. Achenbach, R. Fahrig, J. Hornegger, and A. Maier. "Torsional Heart Motion in Cone-beam Computed Tomography Reconstruction". In: M. King, S. Glick, and K. Mueller, Eds., *Proc. 13th Intl. Mtg. on Fully Three-Dimensional Image Reconstruction in Radiology and Nuclear Medicine*, pp. 651–654, Newport, RI, USA, May 2015.

[Unse 99] M. Unser. "Splines: A Perfect Fit for Signal and Image Processing". *IEEE Signal Proc. Mag.*, Vol. 16, No. 6, pp. 22–38, November 1999.

[Wall 09] M. J. Wallace, M. D. Kuo, C. Glaiberman, C. A. Binkert, R. C. Orth, and G. Soulez. "Three-Dimensional C-arm Cone-beam CT: Applications in the Interventional Suite". *J. Vasc. Interv. Radiol.*, Vol. 20, No. 7, pp. 523–537, July 2009.

[Wein 08] A. Weinlich, B. Keck, H. Scherl, M. Kowarschik, and J. Hornegger. "Comparison of High-Speed Ray Casting on GPU using CUDA and OpenGL". In: *High-performance and Hardware-aware Computing (HipHaC 2008)*, pp. 25–30, Como, Italy, November 2008.

[Wies 00] K. Wiesent, K. Barth, N. Navab, P. Durlak, T. Brunner, O. Schuetz, and W. Seissler. "Enhanced 3-D-reconstruction algorithm for C-arm systems suitable for interventional procedures". *IEEE Trans. Med. Imaging*, Vol. 19, No. 5, pp. 391–403, May 2000.

[Wilk 17] E. Wilkins, L. Wilson, K. Wickramasinghe, P. Bhatnagar, J. Leal, R. Luengo-Fernandez, R. Burns, M. Rayner, and N. Townsend. "European Cardiovascular Disease Statistics 2017". Tech. Rep., European Heart Network, Brussels, Belgium, February 2017.

[Wils 98]   P. Wilson, R. D'Agostino, D. Levy, A. Belanger, H. Silbershatz, and W. Kannel. "Prediction of Coronary Heart Disease Using Risk Factor Categories". *Circulation*, Vol. 97, No. 18, pp. 1837–1847, May 1998.

[Wink 03]   O. Wink, R. Kemkers, S.-Y. Chen, and J. Carroll. "Intra-procedural coronary intervention planning using hybrid 3-dimensional reconstruction techniques". *Acad Radiol*, Vol. 10, No. 12, pp. 1433–1441, December 2003.

[Worl 17]   World Health Organization (WHO). "The top 10 causes of death (Fact sheet No 310)". Online, Jan. 2017.

[Yang 09]   J. Yang, Y. Wang, Y. Liu, S. Tang, and W. Chen. "Novel Approach for 3-D Reconstruction of Coronary Arteries From Two Uncalibrated Angiographic Images". *IEEE Trans. Image Proc.*, Vol. 18, No. 7, pp. 1563–1572, July 2009.

[Yang 12]   G. Yang, Y. Hu, X. Huang, H. Shu, and C. Toumoulin. "Simulation environment of X-ray rotational angiography using 3D+t coronary tree model". In: *Proc. IEEE Eng. Med. Biol. Soc.*, pp. 629–632, IEEE, San Diego, CA, USA, August 2012.

[Yang 14]   J. Yang, W. Cong, Y. Chen, J. Fan, Y. Liu, and Y. Wang. "External force back-projective composition and globally deformable optimization for 3-D coronary artery reconstruction". *Phys. Med. Biol.*, Vol. 59, No. 4, pp. 975–1003, February 2014.

[Zell 05]   M. Zellerhoff, B. Scholz, T. Brunner, and E.-P. Rührnschopf. "Low contrast 3D reconstruction from C-arm data". In: M. Flynn, Ed., *SPIE Medical Imaging: Physics of Medical Imaging*, pp. 646–655, SPIE, San Diego, CA, USA, February 2005.

[Zeng 05]   R. Zeng, J. Fessler, and J. Balter. "Respiratory motion estimation from slowly rotating x-ray projections: Theory and simulation". *Med. Phys.*, Vol. 32, No. 4, pp. 984–991, April 2005.

[Zhu 02]   H. Zhu and M. Friedman. "Tracking 3-D coronary artery motion with biplane angiography". In: *Proc. 2002 IEEE Intl. Symposium on Biomed. Imag. (ISBI)*, pp. 605–608, IEEE, Washington DC, USA, July 2002.

In der Reihe *Studien zur Mustererkennung,*
herausgegeben von
Prof. Dr.-Ing Heinricht Niemann und Herrn Prof. Dr.-Ing. Elmar Nöth
sind bisher erschienen:

9	Volker Warnke	Integrierte Segmentierung und Klassifikation von Äußerungen und Dialogakten mit heterogenen Wissensquellen
		ISBN 978-3-8325-0254-6, 2003, 182 S. 40.50 €
10	Michael Reinhold	Robuste, probabilistische, erscheinungsbasierte Objekterkennung
		ISBN 978-3-8325-0476-2, 2004, 283 S. 40.50 €
11	Matthias Zobel	Optimale Brennweitenwahl für die multiokulare Objektverfolgung
		ISBN 978-3-8325-0496-0, 2004, 292 S. 40.50 €
12	Bernd Ludwig	Ein konfigurierbares Dialogsystem für Mensch-Maschine-Interaktion in gesprochener Sprache
		ISBN 978-3-8325-0497-7, 2004, 230 S. 40.50 €
13	Rainer Deventer	Modeling and Control of Static and Dynamic Systems with Bayesian Networks
		ISBN 978-3-8325-0521-9, 2004, 195 S. 40.50 €
14	Jan Buckow	Multilingual Prosody in Automatic Speech Understanding
		ISBN 978-3-8325-0581-3, 2004, 164 S. 40.50 €
15	Klaus Donath	Automatische Segmentierung und Analyse von Blutgefäßen
		ISBN 978-3-8325-0642-1, 2004, 210 S. 40.50 €
16	Axel Walthelm	Sensorbasierte Lokalisations-Algorithmen für mobile Service-Roboter
		ISBN 978-3-8325-0691-9, 2004, 200 S. 40.50 €
17	Ricarda Dormeyer	Syntaxanalyse auf der Basis der Dependenzgrammatik
		ISBN 978-3-8325-0723-7, 2004, 200 S. 40.50 €
18	Michael Levit	Spoken Language Understanding without Transcriptions in a Call Center Scenario
		ISBN 978-3-8325-0930-9, 2005, 249 S. 40.50 €

29   Andreas Maier   Speech of Children with Cleft Lip and Palate: Automatic Assessment

ISBN 978-3-8325-2144-8, 2009, 220 S.   37.00 €

30   Christian Hacker   Automatic Assessment of Children Speech to Support Language Learning

ISBN 978-3-8325-2258-2, 2009, 272 S.   39.00 €

31   Jan-Henning Trustorff   Der Einsatz von Support Vector Machines zur Kreditwürdigkeitsbeurteilung von Unternehmen

ISBN 978-3-8325-2375-6, 2009, 260 S.   38.00 €

32   Martin Raab   Real World Approaches for Multilingual and Non-native Speech Recognition

ISBN 978-3-8325-2446-3, 2010, 168 S.   44.00 €

33   Michael Wels   Probabilistic Modeling for Segmentation in Magnetic Resonance Images of the Human Brain

ISBN 978-3-8325-2631-3, 2010, 148 S.   40.00 €

34   Florian Jäger   Normalization of Magnetic Resonance Images and its Application to the Diagnosis of the Scoliotic Spine

ISBN 978-3-8325-2779-2, 2011, 168 S.   36.00 €

35   Viktor Zeißler   Robuste Erkennung der prosodischen Phänomene und der emotionalen Benutzerzustände in einem multimodalen Dialogsystem

ISBN 978-3-8325-3167-6, 2012, 380 S.   43.50 €

36   Korbinian Riedhammer   Interactive Approaches to Video Lecture Assessment

ISBN 978-3-8325-3235-2, 2012, 164 S.   40.50 €

37   Stefan Wenhardt   Ansichtenauswahl für die 3-D-Rekonstruktion statischer Szenen

ISBN 978-3-8325-3465-3, 2013, 218 S.   37.00 €

38   Kerstin Müller   3-D Imaging of the Heart Chambers with C-arm CT

ISBN 978-3-8325-3726-5, 2014, 174 S.   46.00 €

48   Chris Schwemmer   3-D Imaging of Coronary Vessels Using C-arm CT

ISBN 978-3-8325-4937-4, 2019, 148 S.   43.50 €

Alle erschienenen Bücher können unter der angegebenen ISBN im Buchhandel oder direkt beim Logos Verlag Berlin (www.logos-verlag.de, Fax: 030 - 42 85 10 92) bestellt werden.